10-Minute
Dog Training Games

QUARRY

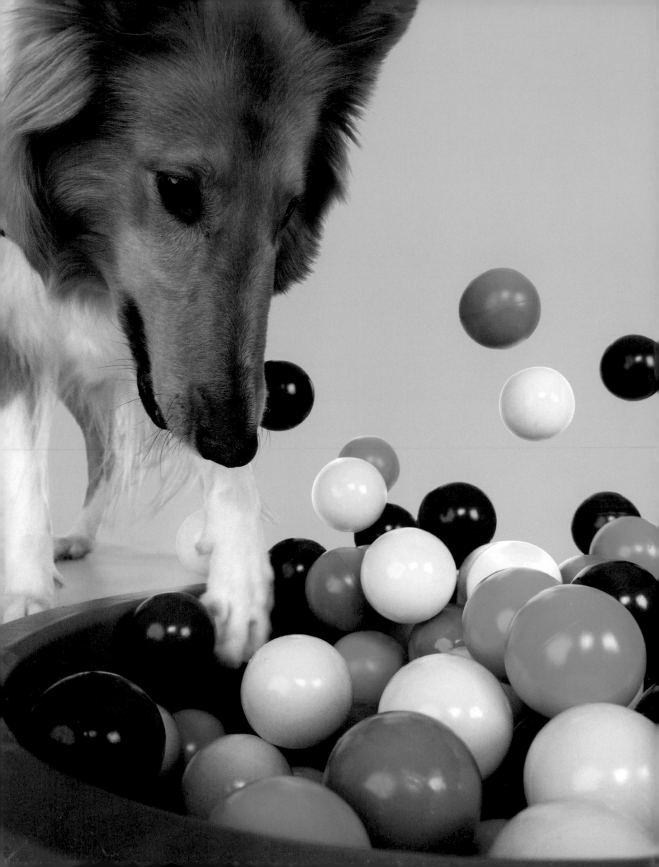

10-Minute
Dog Training Games

Quick and Creative Activities
for the Busy Dog Owner

Kyra Sundance

BEVERLY MASSACHUSETTS

QUARRY BOOKS

© 2011 Quarry Books
Text © 2011 by Kyra Sundance

First published in the United States of America in 2011 by
Quarry Books, a member of
Quayside Publishing Group
100 Cummings Center
Suite 406-L
Beverly, Massachusetts 01915-6101
Telephone: (978) 282-9590
Fax: (978) 283-2742
www.quarrybooks.com

10 9 8 7 6 5 4 3 2 1

ISBN-13: 978-1-59253-730-3

Digital edition published in 2011
eISBN-13: 978-1-61058-156-1

Library of Congress Cataloging-in-Publication Data available

Design: Sundance MediaCom (sundancemediacom.com)
"Do More With Your Dog!" is a registered trademark of
    Kyra Sundance (kyra.com)
Photography: Christian Arias, Slickforce Studios (slickforce.com)

Due to differing conditions, materials, and skill levels, the
publisher and various manufacturers disclaim any liability for
unsatisfactory results or injury due to improper use of tools,
materials, or information.

Printed in Singapore

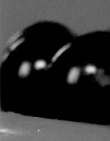

DoMoreWithYourDog.com

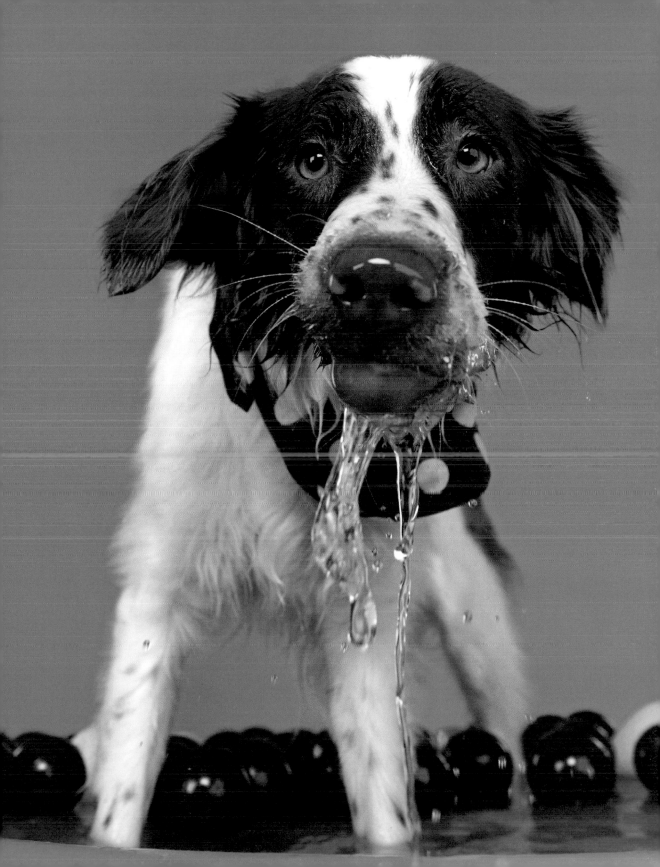

CONTENTS

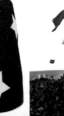

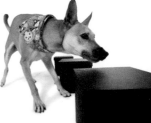

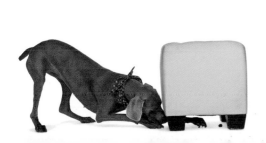
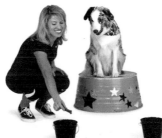
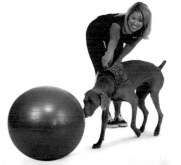

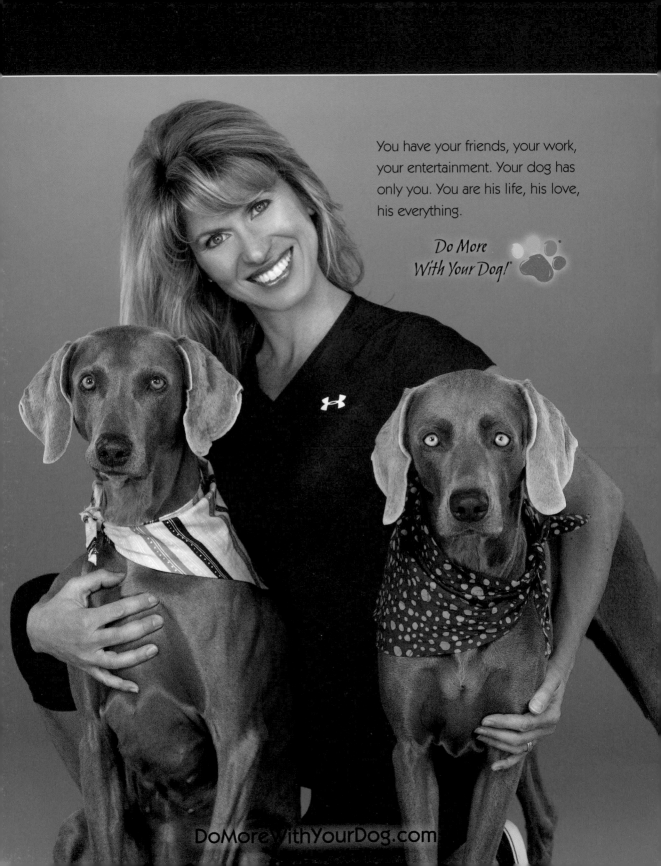

You have your friends, your work, your entertainment. Your dog has only you. You are his life, his love, his everything.

Do More With Your Dog!

Your life is full and busy. You have your friends, your work, your commitments, your hobbies and entertainment.

Your dog has only you. You are his life, his love, his everything. Show him your love in return by setting aside special times with him, in which you give him opportunities for enrichment and your undivided attention.

As a busy dog owner, you want to make the most of the time you have with your dog. The games in this book are structured to provide a mental or physical enrichment exercise that you and your dog can do together. The games are straightforward, and simple enough that your dog can achieve significant success within ten minutes. Working cooperatively with your dog in a positive way will be a wonderful bonding experience, and your dog will bask in your attention and your pride in him. These 10-minute games will be the highlight of his day!

The games in this book are fun activities for your dog, but they are also learning challenges intended to improve your dog's confidence, mental focus, coordination, strength, and ability to follow directions. You can literally see your dog transform from a fearful dog to a water-confident dog after a ten-minute game of Weenie Bobbing (page 14), or from a distracted dog to a focused dog after a ten-minute Memory Game (page 34).

Games will boost the intelligence and cognition of your dog as his brain is challenged with new behaviors. Games benefit puppies as well as senior dogs who still need enrichment and opportunities to feel successful.

I hope this book helps to enhance your relationship, and gives you some new ways to "Do More With Your Dog!®"

Kyra Sundance

Bonds are built through shared experiences: physical, mental, and emotional.

Don't be so focused on the goal that you miss the joys of the journey!

He's YOUR dog, and his success need only be measured in YOUR eyes.

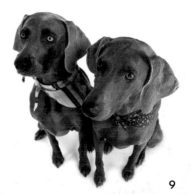

GAMES MAKE A HAPPIER, HEALTHIER DOG

The games in this book are more than fun activities. Each of the games presents a learning challenge for your dog that is intended to improve his confidence, mental focus, coordination, strength, and ability to follow directions. A "teaching skills" box on each game page lists the primary learning opportunities that accompany the game.

These games are intended as a collaborative effort, in which your dog actively works to problem-solve. Refrain from overly controlling your dog, and instead encourage him to experiment. Remember, although these games may look simple to you, they are complex and challenging for your dog.

10 MINUTES!

As a busy dog owner, you try to squeeze in quality time with your dog at every opportunity, even if it is only ten minutes before dinner. The games in this book are structured to provide a significant degree of success within ten minutes. These short, fun sessions are ideal for a dog, and the success he achieves at the end will increase his motivation for training. With over 85 games to choose from, your dog will never bore of training!

TRAINING TIPS

Positive Training Methods

In this book we use positive training methods and a cooperative spirit to build a joyful relationship with your dog in which he is a willing partner in the training process. We instill enthusiasm in the dog by building his esteem and his motivation.

Provide a consistent and motivating environment for your dog as you guide him through each new game. Reward each of his small successes along the way and use your "happy voice" to encourage and praise him.

Reward Success, Ignore the Rest

One of the key skills your dog develops through games is his ability to problem-solve through experimentation. Encourage your dog to try a lot of behaviors and let him know (with a treat) which ones were correct.

When your dog offers a behavior that is not correct, don't say "no," but rather simply ignore his unsuccessful attempt. Saying "no" could discourage your dog and make him reluctant to try anything at all.

Food Treats

Although a reward for a dog can be a toy, play, or praise, we usually use food treats because they are a high-value reward and can be dispensed quickly. During the learning stages of a new game, you want to make it very rewarding for your dog by giving lots of treats for every small success. In fact, you may give your dog his entire dinner, piece by piece, during a ten-minute game.

Keep your dog extra motivated by using "people food" treats, such as pea-size pieces of chicken, steak, cheese, goldfish crackers, noodles, or meatballs. Try microwaving hot dog slices on a paper-towel-covered plate for three minutes for a tasty treat!

Calming an Overly Excited Dog

Sometimes a dog becomes so excited during a game that you need to get him to calm down and regain focus. Do this by silently putting your arms at your sides and looking away for a few seconds. This will inform your dog (without reprimanding or frustrating him) that he is not on a path that will lead to a reward, and he needs to give you his calm attention. A few seconds is usually enough for him calm down a bit, at which time you can resume the game. Repeat this process every time your dog gets too hyper.

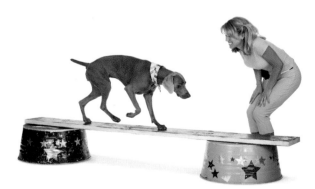

Lure, Don't Manipulate

There are two obvious ways to get a dog into a desired position: You can lure him by encouraging him to follow a treat, or you can physically manipulate him into position. It is tempting to manipulate your dog's body physically; however, it can actually delay the learning process, as the dog is not required to engage his brain and is not learning the motor skills necessary to position his body himself. It is always preferable to lure your dog to position his body himself.

Timing

During the learning process, your dog may squirm and try a variety of different things. You need to let him know immediately if each thing he tried was a success (treat) or nonsuccess (no treat). The key to helping him understand the goal behavior is to give him the treat at the exact moment that he performed correctly. Be ready with a treat in your hand and release it the instant your dog performs correctly. Don't reward five seconds after he has done the behavior, as your dog may not understand what he did to earn the reward.

Marker Training

It can sometimes be logistically difficult to reward your dog at the exact moment he performed correctly. But you *can* use a specific word (or a clicker) at that exact moment to let your dog know the instant he earned his reward. We call this special sound a **reward marker** because it marks the instant your dog earned a reward. A reward marker is always quickly followed by a treat. Some trainers use a reward marker of "good!" or "yes!"

Regression Is Part of Progression

The key to keeping your dog motivated is to keep him challenged and achieving regular successes. If your dog goes for thirty seconds without getting a treat, he could become discouraged and not wish to continue. If your dog is struggling, temporarily lower the criteria for success. Regress back to an easier step where he can be successful for a while.

Your dog will go through spurts of learning and regression. Don't be reluctant to go back a step—it's usually only needed for a short while and will give your dog confidence to move forward.

HOW TO USE THIS BOOK

Start anywhere! Each game displays an "equipment" box that will give you instruction on constructing the needed equipment. Once you've finished with a game, a "build on it" box will point you toward another game that utilizes your dog's newly learned skill.

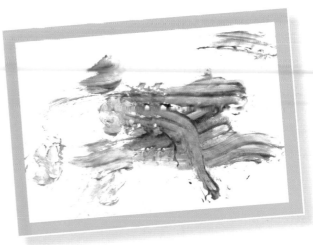

"Horse and Rider"
by Holly, Alaskan malamute, 2010

The paper was oriented vertically when Holly painted it, and Holly's owner was surprised to see the picture when she rotated it. Holly painted this picture days after her infamous stunt in which she bolted from the obedience competition ring and into the adjoining field, where she chased the ponies in the middle of their televised polo match.

Try Pawprint Painting with your dog, page 170.

GAMES ARE A FOUNDATION FOR DOG SPORTS

Many of the games in this book are used by top trainers as foundation skills for dog sports. They introduce the dog to the body awareness and logic skills that he will need in his sport. On every game page in this book you will find a box listing the primary sports and activities that utilize this game as a training skill. Below are brief descriptions of some common dog sports that are referenced in this book.

Agility

Dog agility is one of the most popular dog sports. In this race the dog, guided by his handler, maneuvers through a path of obstacles including jumps, seesaws, weave poles, tire jumps, A-frames, dogwalks (elevated planks), tunnels, and pause tables. In every competition, obstacles are arranged in a different order within a roughly 100 x 100-foot (30 x 30 m) course. One dog and handler run the course at a time, competing for the fastest time. The handler guides her dog with verbal commands and body language. Fault deductions occur for mistakes such as jumping off the seesaw without touching the yellow bottom portion of it (called the contact zone).

Lure Coursing

Lure coursing is a high-energy sport in which dogs chase a mechanically operated artificial lure (such as a white plastic bag or tanned rabbit skins). The lure is attached to a string that is pulled by a motor around the course, with pulleys to create turns. The lure travels at speeds up to 40 miles (64 km) per hour.

Nose Work

This recreational and titling sport uses a dog's natural abilities to hunt for and locate a target odor. Inspired by the work of police detection K-9s, dog and handler teams have fun searching boxes for a hidden scented object. It's a great way for a dog to have fun, build confidence, and burn mental and physical energy.

Tracking

As part of their hunting instinct, all dogs have the ability to track, or follow a scent trail. Dogs can be trained to follow the path traversed by a person. Tracking trials (competitions) emulate the search for a missing person. A tracklayer walks through a field. The dog and handler then start at one end of the track and try to follow it to the end.

Search and Rescue

Trained volunteer search and rescue (SAR) dog/handler teams assist in law enforcement requests to search for missing people, such as people lost in the wilderness or trapped by an avalanche. Dogs are trained to track scent trails and to use their noses to find people.

Flying Disc

In disc toss-and-fetch competition the handler and dog work as a team to make as many successful throws/catches as they can during a timed round. In freestyle disc competition, dog and handler execute high-skill disc tricks in a choreographed routine set to music. It may include flips, multiple catches, and body vaults, making this a popular event with spectators.

Field Retrieving

Field hunting dogs are used to retrieve downed birds. Retriever hunting tests provide a way to demonstrate your dog's retrieving instinct and training and to earn titles. The handler directs his dog to a downed bird by using whistles and arm signals. The handler whistles to command his dog to sit and look at him. He then extends an arm to his right or left to indicate the direction he wishes his dog is to travel.

Rally-O

In rally-o (also called rally obedience or rally) dog and handler teams navigate a course of ten to twenty numbered stations, each with a sign indicating a behavior to perform at that station such as "halt and sit," "U-turn," "moving down," or "call dog front and finish left." This is a self-guided course in which the handler proceeds with her dog at heel, at her own pace, through each station. Unlike in traditional obedience, handlers are allowed to encourage, praise, and double command their dogs through the course.

Obedience Competition

In competition dog obedience you and your dog work as a team to earn titles and rankings. Each competition level consists of six or seven defined exercises that are scored by a judge. Novice-level exercises consist of things like heeling, figure-8 heeling, recall ("come"), stand for examination, sit-stay, and down-stay.

Schutzhund

Schutzhund (meaning *protection dog*) tests a dog for the traits necessary for police-type work such as police K-9, odor/drug detection, tracking, and search and rescue. The dog must demonstrate courage, intelligence, trainability, and a desire to work, as well as physical strength, endurance, agility, and scenting ability. Schutzhund trials (tests) consist of three phases: tracking, obedience, and protection.

Musical Canine Freestyle

Musical canine freestyle (also called dog dancing) is a choreographed routine by a dog and handler, set to music. Competition showcases dance ability, creativity, and innovative dog tricks. Moves may include leg weaves, figure-8s through the handler's legs, jumps, spins, bows, rolls, and leg kicks.

Conformation Dog Show

Conformation dog show is the most popular form of canine competition. Every breed has a recognized breed standard representing its ideal characteristics. A dog show judge compares each dog to his breed standard to find the dog nearest to that ideal. The dog is judged on his conformation (overall appearance and structure). Dogs are lined up and stacked (positioned squarely and evenly so that the judge can evaluate their structure) and then gaited around the ring. Mixed-breed dogs can compete in companion dog shows, in which the handler's skill at presenting the dog is evaluated but not the dog's physical structure.

Animal Actor

Dog actors are used in movies, on TV, in commercials, and in live shows. Many dog actors are privately owned and contracted through animal talent agencies. They must be confident and well socialized to people, environments, and loud noises. They also must be set-trained and able to perform basic behaviors on cue with silent hand-signal cues.

Therapy Dog

Volunteering as a certified therapy dog team is a rewarding way to share your dog and bring smiles to the faces of people you visit by visiting them in hospitals or other facilities and providing comfort and a friendly distraction from stress or pain. A therapy dog must be confident and well socialized. Some dogs contribute to the visiting experience by performing simple tricks.

Service Dog

A service dog (also called an assistance dog) is specially trained to help a person with a particular disability. Assist dogs may be trained to pull a wheelchair, pick things up from the floor, open and close doors, or pull a seated person to a standing position. Some dogs are trained to hit a special button that phones emergency services.

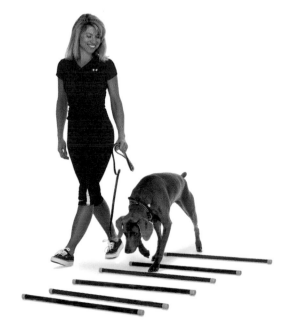

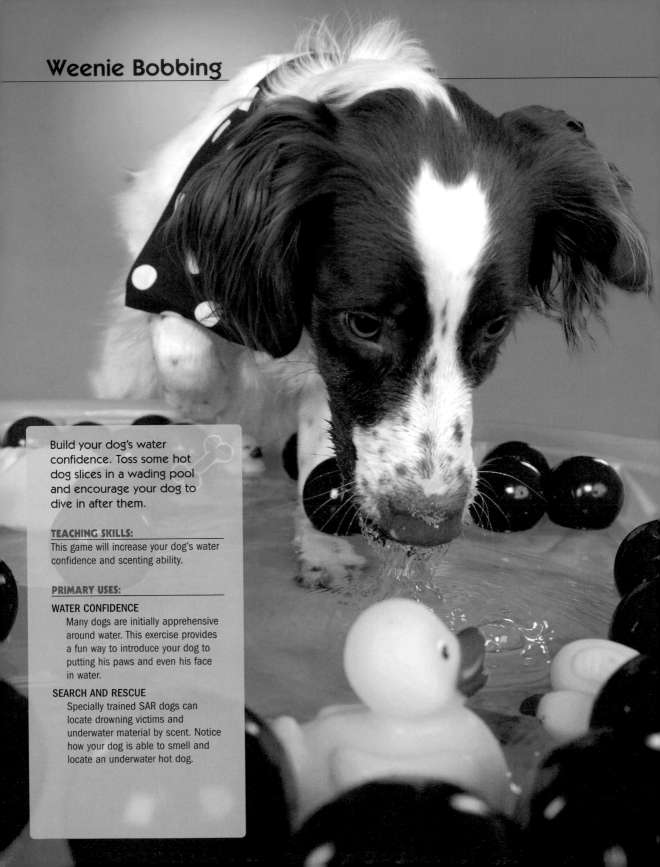

Weenie Bobbing

Build your dog's water confidence. Toss some hot dog slices in a wading pool and encourage your dog to dive in after them.

TEACHING SKILLS:
This game will increase your dog's water confidence and scenting ability.

PRIMARY USES:

WATER CONFIDENCE
Many dogs are initially apprehensive around water. This exercise provides a fun way to introduce your dog to putting his paws and even his face in water.

SEARCH AND RESCUE
Specially trained SAR dogs can locate drowning victims and underwater material by scent. Notice how your dog is able to smell and locate an underwater hot dog.

TRY IT:

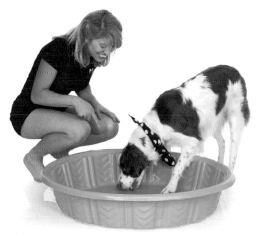

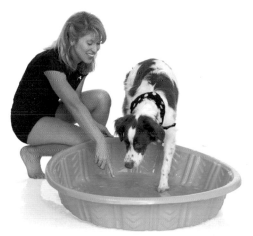

1 Show your dog that you're tossing a few hot dog slices into an empty wading pool. Toss at least one hot dog close enough to the edge so that your dog can get it without stepping into the pool. Keep encouraging your dog until he has the confidence to step into the empty pool.

2 Add just an inch of water to the wading pool and repeat the exercise. Praise your dog for any advances he makes. If your dog is reluctant, place the wading pool on a slight slope so that the upper half of the pool is dry.

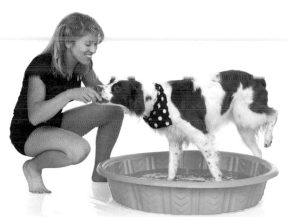

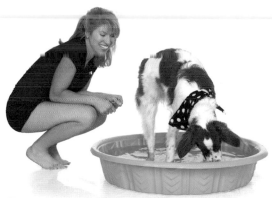

3 Add more water to the pool and encourage your dog to jump in with all four feet! Use a treat in your hand to get him to walk through the water.

4 Some dogs learn to "dive" for treats and can pick them up from the bottom of the pool. They even blow bubbles from their nose when they submerge their faces.

TIP:

It is important that you don't push your dog toward a feared object but instead allow him to approach it on his own. Pushing your dog or physically placing him in the wading pool can increase his fear and set training back considerably. Within ten minutes, most dogs are happily sloshing after the hot dogs!

EQUIPMENT:

Use a child's wading pool, a large water bucket, or even a large bowl for this game.

BUILD ON IT:

Hunt in Box of Packing Material
page 16

Body Board
page 96

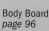

Hunt in Box of Packing Material

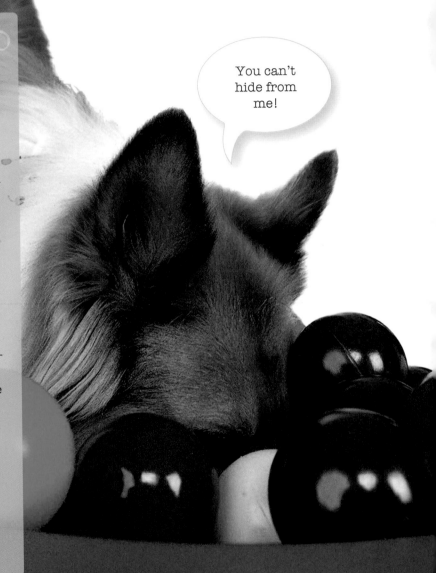

Hide a treat or toy in a box of packing material. Your dog will gain confidence (and have fun) as he burrows in after it!

TEACHING SKILLS:

This game builds confidence, scenting ability, mental focus, and independent hunting skills.

PRIMARY USES:

NOSE WORK

This game introduces your dog to searching for an object by scent.

SEARCH AND RESCUE

SAR dogs are trained to search for people by scent and to confidently follow that scent through debris such as building rubble. This game builds such confidence and perseverance in your dog.

TRY IT:

Get your dog interested in a treat or favorite toy. Make sure he is watching as you place it just barely under the surface of the packing material. Point to it, tap it, and encourage your dog in an excited voice to "get it!" When he does, act very excited and let him have the treat or toy as his reward.

You can't hide from me!

TIP:

Your dog may be apprehensive at first and reluctant to bury his head in the packing material. Over time he will gain confidence and persistence, and you can bury the item deeper.

EQUIPMENT:

Fill a box with packing material such as nontoxic packing peanuts, wadded-up newspaper balls, or child's ball-pit balls. Put the treat inside a treat bag or ventilated container to make it a larger target for your dog.

BUILD ON IT:

Muffin Tin
page 46

Laundry Basket

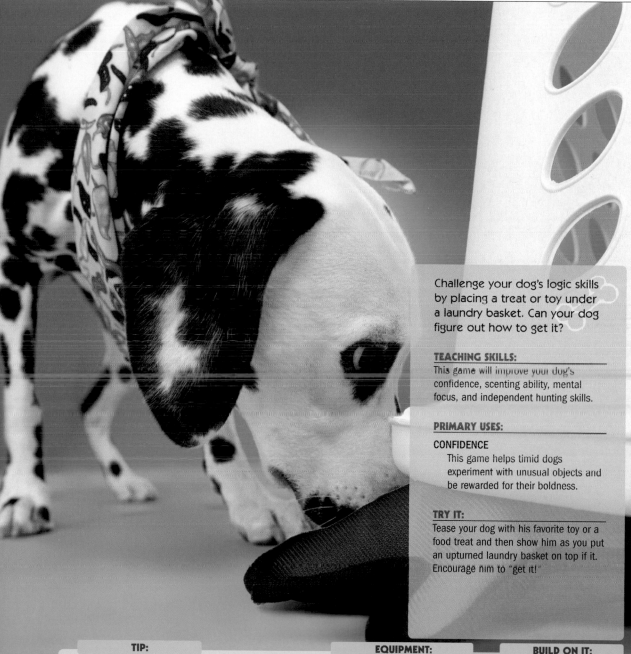

Challenge your dog's logic skills by placing a treat or toy under a laundry basket. Can your dog figure out how to get it?

TEACHING SKILLS:
This game will improve your dog's confidence, scenting ability, mental focus, and independent hunting skills.

PRIMARY USES:

CONFIDENCE
This game helps timid dogs experiment with unusual objects and be rewarded for their boldness.

TRY IT:
Tease your dog with his favorite toy or a food treat and then show him as you put an upturned laundry basket on top if it. Encourage him to "get it!"

TIP:
Your dog will learn to enjoy this game . . . but only if he experiences success in the beginning stages. You don't want your dog to give up and walk away, so when he shows interest in the basket by nosing or pawing it, help him by slightly lifting a corner of the basket.

EQUIPMENT:
Use a wire or plastic laundry basket with holes large enough for your dog to see and smell the treat underneath.

BUILD ON IT:

Tied-Up Towel
page 47

Tunnel

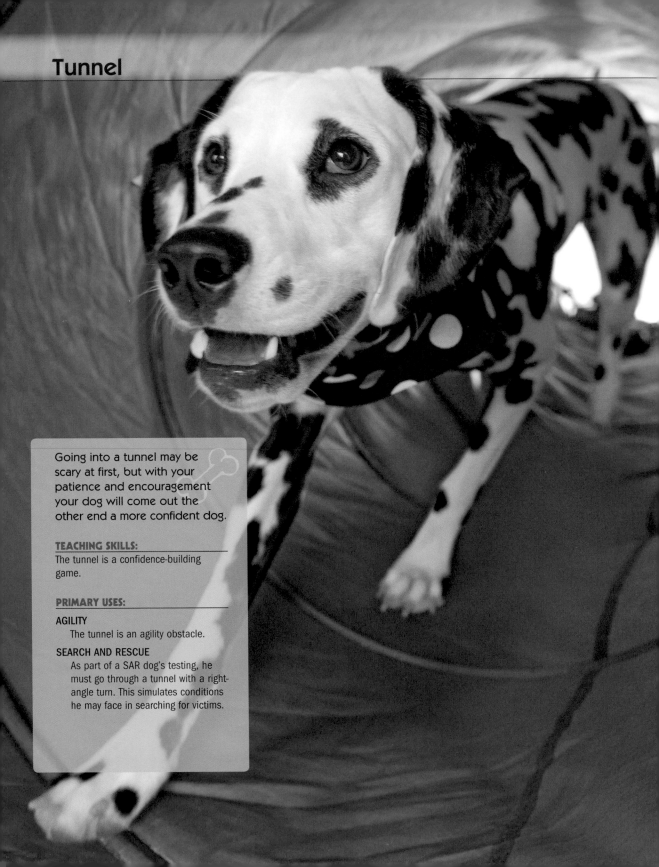

Going into a tunnel may be scary at first, but with your patience and encouragement your dog will come out the other end a more confident dog.

TEACHING SKILLS:
The tunnel is a confidence-building game.

PRIMARY USES:

AGILITY
The tunnel is an agility obstacle.

SEARCH AND RESCUE
As part of a SAR dog's testing, he must go through a tunnel with a right-angle turn. This simulates conditions he may face in searching for victims.

TRY IT:

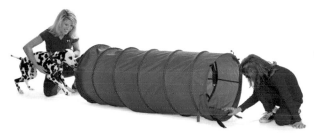
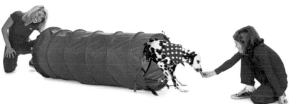

1 Allow your dog time to explore a short, straight tunnel in a familiar area. Have someone hold your dog at one end of the tunnel while you call your dog and make eye contact with him from the other end. Extend a treat into the tunnel to coax him toward you.

2 It may take several minutes or more of coaxing . . . be patient. When your dog finally goes through the tunnel, give him the treat.

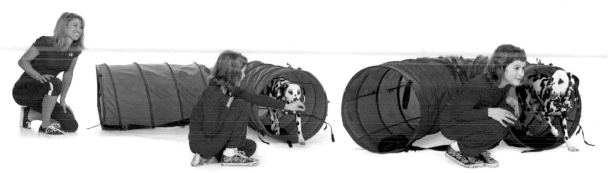

3 Once your dog is confident running through a straight tunnel, try putting a slight bend in it. Don't be surprised if your dog becomes once again apprehensive. You may need to have him go through a straight tunnel a few times to give him confidence before trying the bent tunnel again.

4 Make it even more challenging for your dog by putting a full U-turn bend in the tunnel. Calling to your dog as he runs through the tunnel will let him hear where you are, and give him confidence.

TIP:

Once accustomed to it, most dogs really enjoy running through the tunnel. If you don't have someone to help hold your dog at the entrance of the tunnel, set the tunnel between a wall and a sofa, or in a doorway, so your dog cannot go around the tunnel.

EQUIPMENT:

Competition agility tunnels are 24 inches (61 cm) in diameter; however, smaller, children's tunnels can be purchased at a significantly lower price. Use sand bags inside the tunnel to hold it steady.

BUILD ON IT:

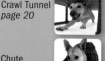
Crawl Tunnel
page 20

Chute
page 22

Crawl Tunnel

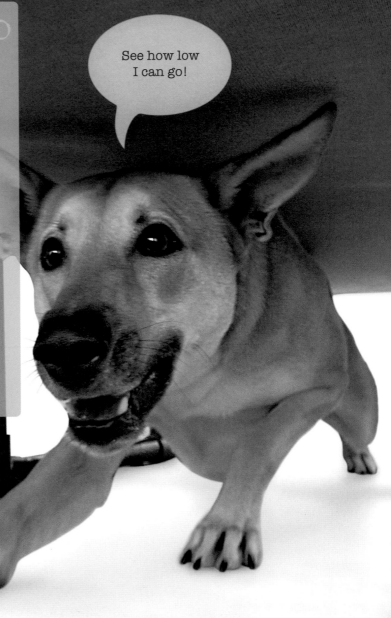

Gradually lower the tunnel ceiling until your dog is belly crawling under it.

TEACHING SKILLS:

This game will increase your dog's confidence and strength. The crawl tunnel is sometimes used in the rehabilitation of injuries.

PRIMARY USES:

AGILITY

The crawl tunnel obstacle is used in some agility trials.

SEARCH AND RESCUE / POLICE K-9

SAR and police K-9 units use crawl tunnels to teach their dogs to maneuver under tight places—a skill which may be needed when the dog is searching for someone or is sent to retrieve an object. A SAR dog must be able to crawl under an obstacle that is three-quarters of the dog's height.

See how low I can go!

TRY IT:

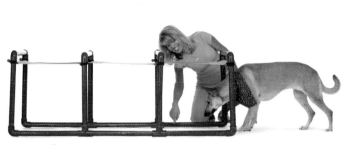

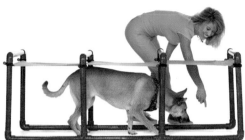

1 Adjust the crawl tunnel ceiling to its highest height. Set it against a wall so that your dog cannot come out the side. Place a line of treats through the tunnel. Bring your dog to the tunnel entrance and point out the first treat to him. Position your body on the side of the tunnel to discourage your dog from coming out the side.

2 After eating the first treat, your dog may back out of the tunnel entrance. Allow him to do so, and simply put another treat in the same spot. Try adding more treats in the tunnel and space them closer together to keep him moving forward. Soon he should be comfortable going all the way through. Repeat the exercise in the opposite direction.

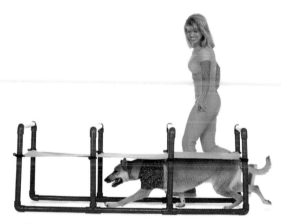

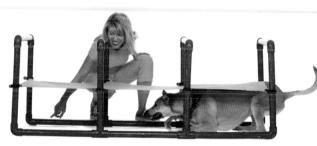

3 Move the tunnel away from the wall and speed your pace as you walk alongside of the tunnel. Lower the ceiling in small increments.

4 Incorporate your cue word, "crawl." Your dog will be much more willing to crawl on a comfortable surface such as grass or carpet. Crawling is hard work for a dog, so do only a few repetitions.

TIP:	**EQUIPMENT:**	**BUILD ON IT:**
Your dog may be initially fearful of the crawl tunnel, so it is important that you don't push him past his comfort level, as this could increase his fear. Allow him to maneuver through the tunnel on his own terms and be able to escape when he wants to.	Agility crawl tunnels are 75 inches (2 m) long by 33 inches (84 cm) wide. You can make a crawl tunnel by extending the legs of a dog ladder (page 68). You can even improvise a crawl tunnel by lining up several sawhorses or chairs for your dog to crawl under.	Chute page 22

Chute

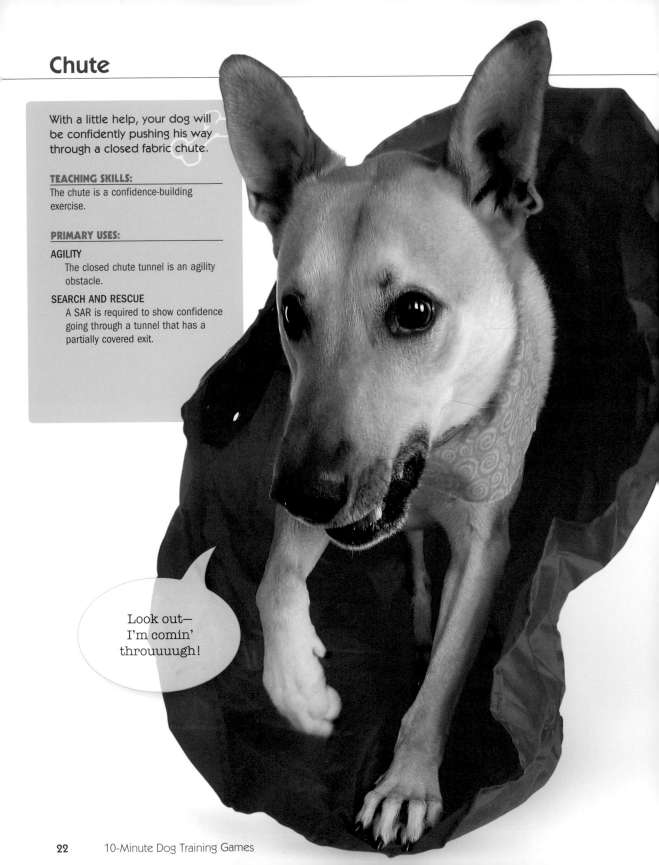

With a little help, your dog will be confidently pushing his way through a closed fabric chute.

TEACHING SKILLS:
The chute is a confidence-building exercise.

PRIMARY USES:

AGILITY
The closed chute tunnel is an agility obstacle.

SEARCH AND RESCUE
A SAR is required to show confidence going through a tunnel that has a partially covered exit.

Look out—
I'm comin'
throuuuugh!

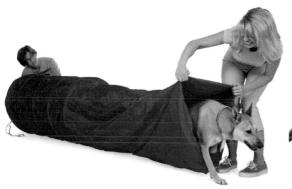 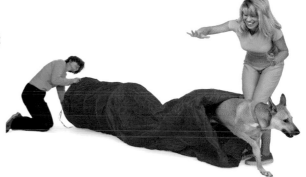

1 First, teach your dog to go through an open Tunnel (page 18). Have a helper hold your dog at the chute tunnel entrance. Stand at the exit and lift open the fabric chute so your dog can see all the way through. Call your dog through and give him a treat when he exits.

2 Try it again, but this time drop the fabric chute on top of your dog just as he is exiting, so that he gets used to the fabric touching his body.

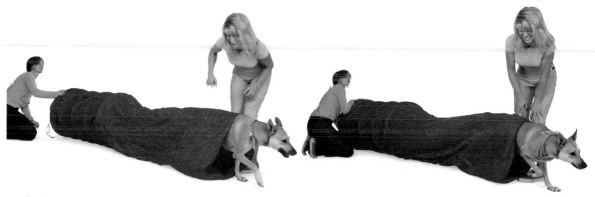

3 Now drop the fabric even sooner, so that your dog has to push his way through the last few feet.

4 Lift up the fabric so your dog can see all the way through, and then drop the fabric back down to the floor. Immediately call your dog through. Congratulate him for his bravery!

TIP:	EQUIPMENT:	BUILD ON IT:
Straighten the fabric chute before every run so your dog does not get tangled inside. If your dog does get tangled do not grab your dog, but rather lift and expand the opening of the chute.	Agility chute tunnels come in a variety of qualities and prices. Improvise a chute by attaching a garbage bag to a 55-gallon (208 L) plastic barrel, or by simply draping a blanket over a table for your dog to push through.	Blind Jump *page 32*

Bang Game

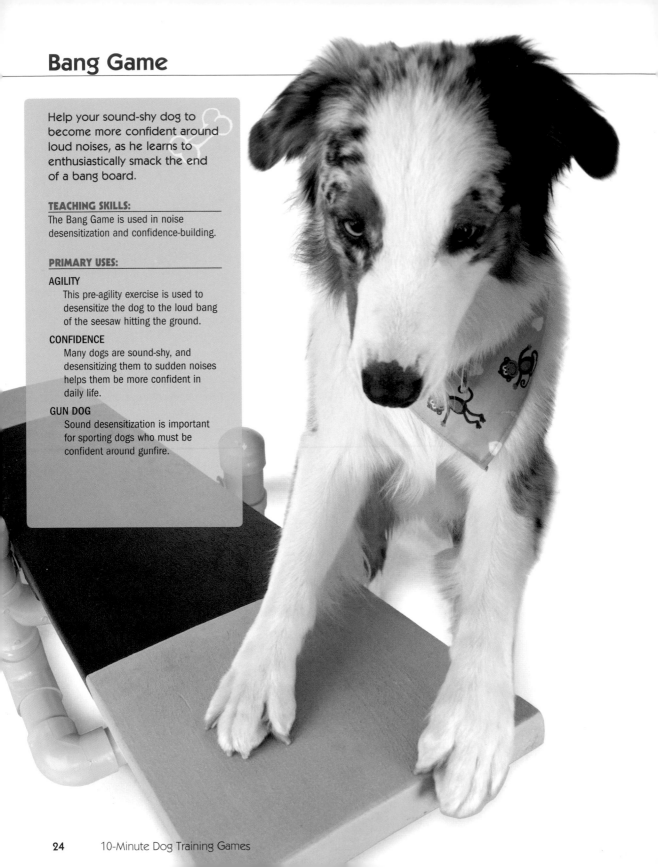

Help your sound-shy dog to become more confident around loud noises, as he learns to enthusiastically smack the end of a bang board.

TEACHING SKILLS:

The Bang Game is used in noise desensitization and confidence-building.

PRIMARY USES:

AGILITY

This pre-agility exercise is used to desensitize the dog to the loud bang of the seesaw hitting the ground.

CONFIDENCE

Many dogs are sound-shy, and desensitizing them to sudden noises helps them be more confident in daily life.

GUN DOG

Sound desensitization is important for sporting dogs who must be confident around gunfire.

TRY IT:

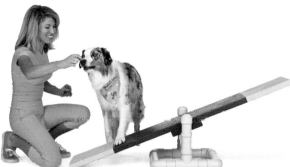

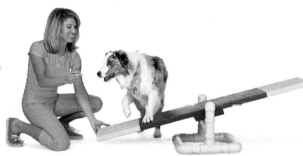

1 Hold a treat above the downward end of the bang board and tell your dog, "Paws up!" As your dog reaches for the treat, he may try to step on the board. As soon as a paw comes on the board, say, "Good!" and give him the treat.

2 Hold the end of the bang board an inch (3 cm) above the ground and repeat the exercise. When your dog steps on the board, allow it to drop to the ground. Your dog may be startled by its movement and noise, so keep your praise happy and encouraging.

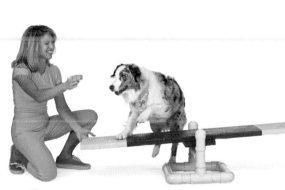

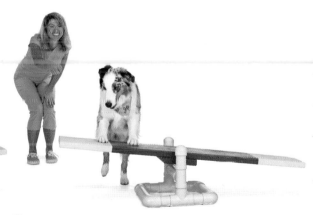

3 Gradually hold the end of the bang board higher. Reward every bang with happy praise and a treat. If your dog seems unsure, go back to putting the board all the way to the ground for a few tries.

4 Let your dog do it on his own. When your dog starts his agility training, he will already be desensitized to the scary bang of the seesaw obstacle.

TIP:

Counterconditioning is a technique that pairs a reward (treat) with a feared object (the loud bang) to overcome the fear. Be cognizant of your dog's anxiety level and work below his fear threshold. If your dog is crouching, reluctant to approach the bang board, or does not take your food treat, then he is over that threshold.

EQUIPMENT:

Bang boards look like mini seesaws. You can also use a full sized seesaw (page 88) or wobble board (page 94) as your "bang" object.

BUILD ON IT:

Slam the Door
page 26

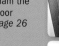

Seesaw
page 88

Slam the Door

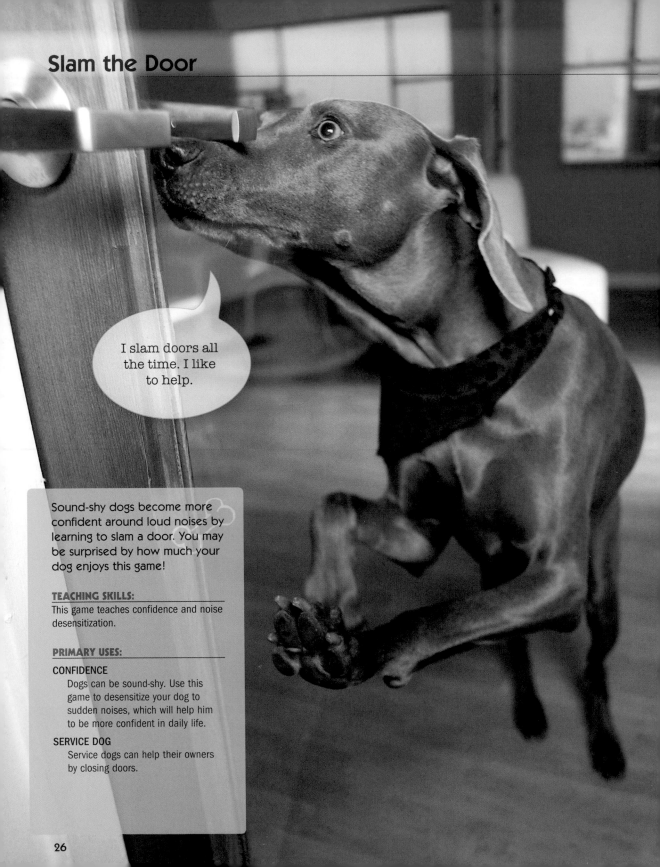

I slam doors all the time. I like to help.

Sound-shy dogs become more confident around loud noises by learning to slam a door. You may be surprised by how much your dog enjoys this game!

TEACHING SKILLS:
This game teaches confidence and noise desensitization.

PRIMARY USES:

CONFIDENCE
Dogs can be sound-shy. Use this game to desensitize your dog to sudden noises, which will help him to be more confident in daily life.

SERVICE DOG
Service dogs can help their owners by closing doors.

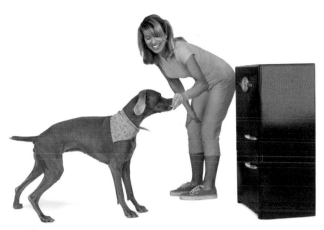

1 Start with a door that is already closed. Hold a treat to your dog's nose to get him interested.

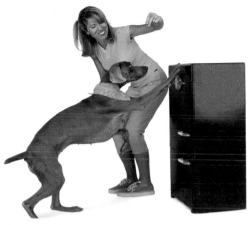

2 Slowly move the treat toward the door, and up to a height that is just out of your dog's reach. In an attempt to get the treat, your dog will put his front paws on the door. At that instant, say, "Good!" and give him the treat.

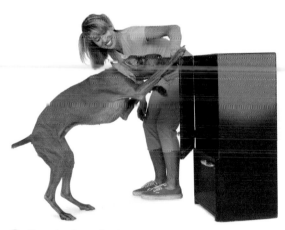

3 Open the door a few inches and repeat the exercise. When your dog puts his paws on the door, the door will slam, which may startle your dog. As quickly as possible after the slam, get that treat into your dog's mouth.

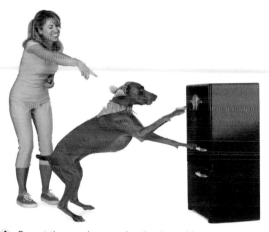

4 Repeat the exercise, opening the door wider as your dog gains confidence. Soon, your dog will be excitedly jumping against the door to make it slam!

TIP:	EQUIPMENT:	BUILD ON IT:
A sound-shy dog will startle at the loud slamming sound, so it is important to increase the noise level gradually. Be cognizant of your dog's anxiety level. If he is reluctant to approach the door, go back to practicing with a closed door.	Use a door for larger dogs, and a kitchen cabinet for small dogs.	Ring a Bell to Go Out *page 152* Pawprint Painting *page 170*

Hoop Jump

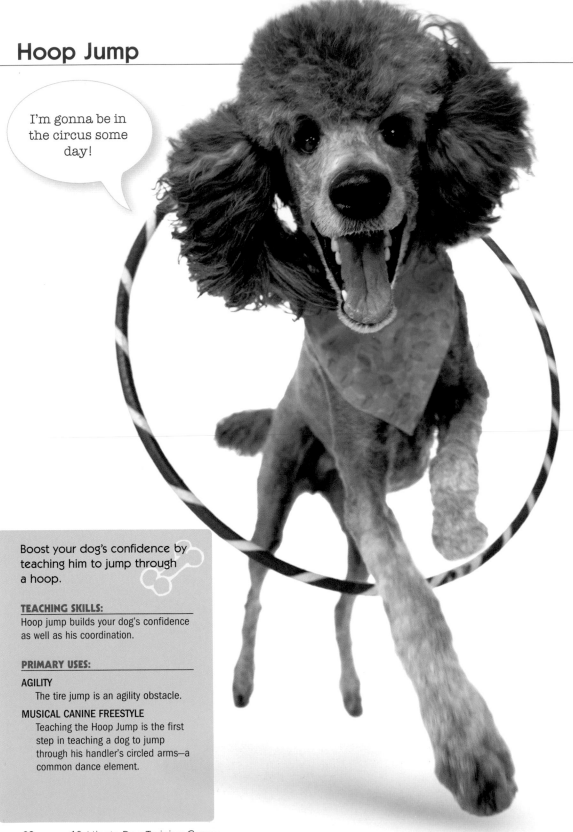

I'm gonna be in the circus some day!

Boost your dog's confidence by teaching him to jump through a hoop.

TEACHING SKILLS:
Hoop jump builds your dog's confidence as well as his coordination.

PRIMARY USES:

AGILITY
The tire jump is an agility obstacle.

MUSICAL CANINE FREESTYLE
Teaching the Hoop Jump is the first step in teaching a dog to jump through his handler's circled arms—a common dance element.

TRY IT:

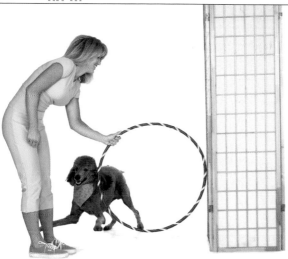

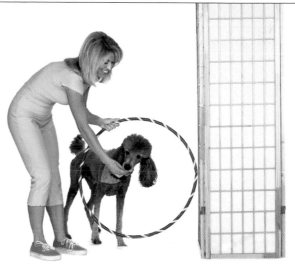

1 Hold the hoop across a doorway so that your dog will not be able to go around the hoop. Give your dog some time to investigate the hoop, as he may be scared of it at first.

2 Use the hand closer to your dog to hold the hoop. In your other hand, hold a treat and lure your dog through the hoop. Let him have the treat once he goes through.

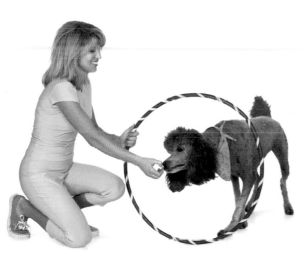

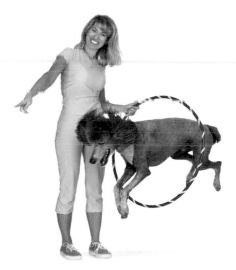

3 Now try it in an open room. Hold the hoop on the ground using the hand closer to your dog. Say, "Hup!" and lure him through with a treat in your other hand.

4 Raise the hoop off the floor. Use the hand opposite your dog to wave energetically. If your dog gets tangled in the hoop, be ready to release it.

TIP:	EQUIPMENT:	BUILD ON IT:
Dogs can be frightened to go through the hoop for the first time. Allow your dog to make the decision to go through on his own, without forcing him.	Remove the noisy beads from inside a toy hoop, as they may frighten your dog. Or make your own hoop from black PVC irrigation tubing and tubing connectors (sold at home improvement stores).	Bar Jump page 104

Platform Jump

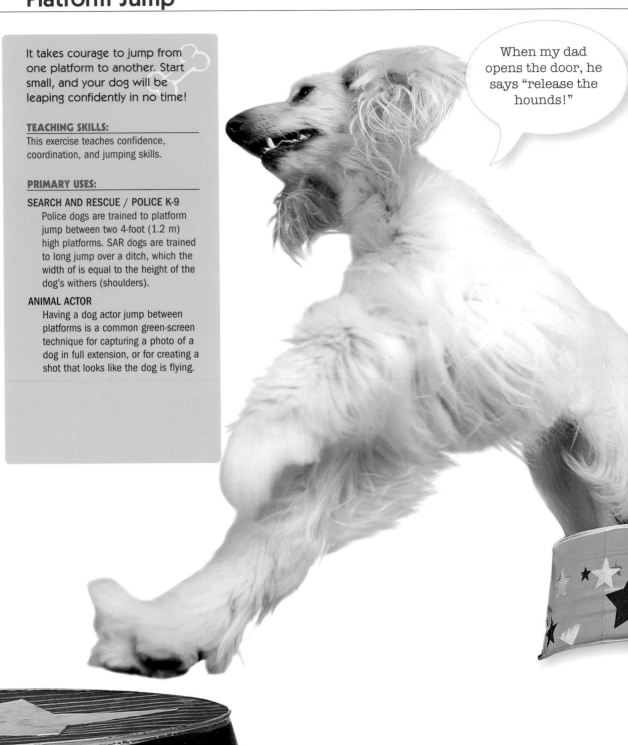

It takes courage to jump from one platform to another. Start small, and your dog will be leaping confidently in no time!

TEACHING SKILLS:

This exercise teaches confidence, coordination, and jumping skills.

PRIMARY USES:

SEARCH AND RESCUE / POLICE K-9

Police dogs are trained to platform jump between two 4-foot (1.2 m) high platforms. SAR dogs are trained to long jump over a ditch, which the width of is equal to the height of the dog's withers (shoulders).

ANIMAL ACTOR

Having a dog actor jump between platforms is a common green-screen technique for capturing a photo of a dog in full extension, or for creating a shot that looks like the dog is flying.

When my dad opens the door, he says "release the hounds!"

TRY IT:

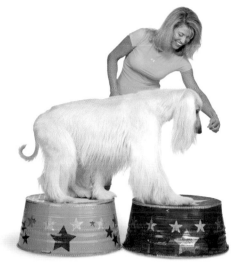

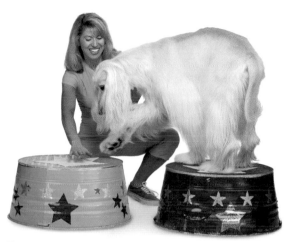

1 Set up two adjoining platforms. Have your dog "step up" onto the first platform (see Pedestal, page 136). Use a treat to lure him onto the second platform. Give him the treat when he reaches the second platform.

2 Separate the platforms by about 6 inches (15 cm) and try it again. Instead of luring your dog to the second platform, try saying, "Hup!" and patting it.

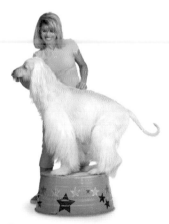

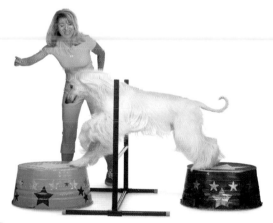

3 Gradually separate the platforms so that your dog is jumping farther distances. Always reward your dog on the second platform.

4 If your dog jumps to the ground instead of the second platform, place a bar jump or hoop between the two platforms.

TIP:	EQUIPMENT:	BUILD ON IT:
A bad experience with a jump can decrease your dog's confidence, so increase the distances very slowly, and only when you are sure your dog feels confident.	Platforms should be sturdy with good traction, and large enough to provide adequate landing space for your dog (the farther apart the platforms, the larger the platforms will need to be). There is always the possibility that your dog will fall short on his jump, so use platforms low enough that your dog will not get hurt if he falls short (approximately half of the height of your dog).	Bar Jump *page 104*

Blind Jump

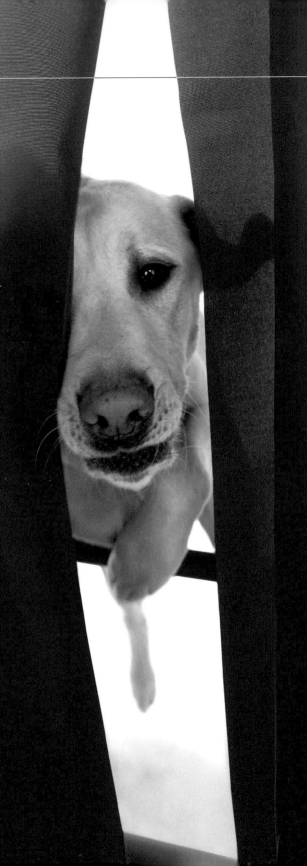

It's empowering for a dog to conquer his fears. With your encouragement, your dog can be confidently jumping through a closed curtain.

TEACHING SKILLS:
A Blind Jump teaches confidence as well as jumping skills.

PRIMARY USES:

AGILITY
The blind jump is similar to the "window jump" agility obstacle. This obstacle consists of a solid fabric panel with a square window cutout. As with the blind jump, the dog cannot see what is on the other side of the window jump.

SEARCH AND RESCUE / POLICE K-9
SAR and police K-9s are trained on a window jump obstacle to prepare for a scenario in which they may need to jump through an actual window.

TRY IT:

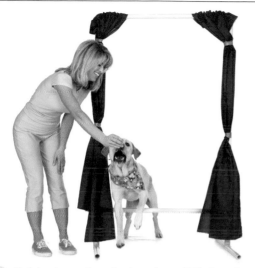

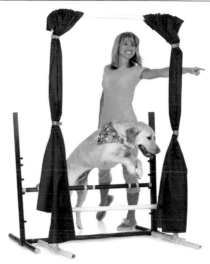

1 First, teach your dog a Bar Jump (page 104). Open the curtains on your blind jump all the way and tie them to the sides of the frame so they don't move in the breeze. Use a treat to lure your dog through the frame.

2 Set up a low bar jump directly in front of your blind jump, and have your dog jump over the bar and through the blind jump frame.

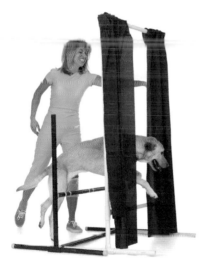

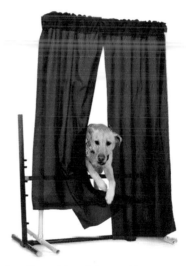

3 Untie the curtains, but keep them open. Have your dog jump over the bar and through the blind jump. After each jump, close the curtains a little more.

4 Finally, close the curtains all the way. There should still be a small sliver of an opening so that your dog knows where to jump.

TIP:	EQUIPMENT:	BUILD ON IT:
Work each step of this exercise and don't progress too fast. Mastering this skill will lead to a more confident dog.	Construct a PVC plastic pipe frame for your blind jump. Attach a split curtain made from lightweight fabric. Improvise a blind jump by simply attaching fabric or newspaper to a large hoop.	Chute page 22

Memory Game

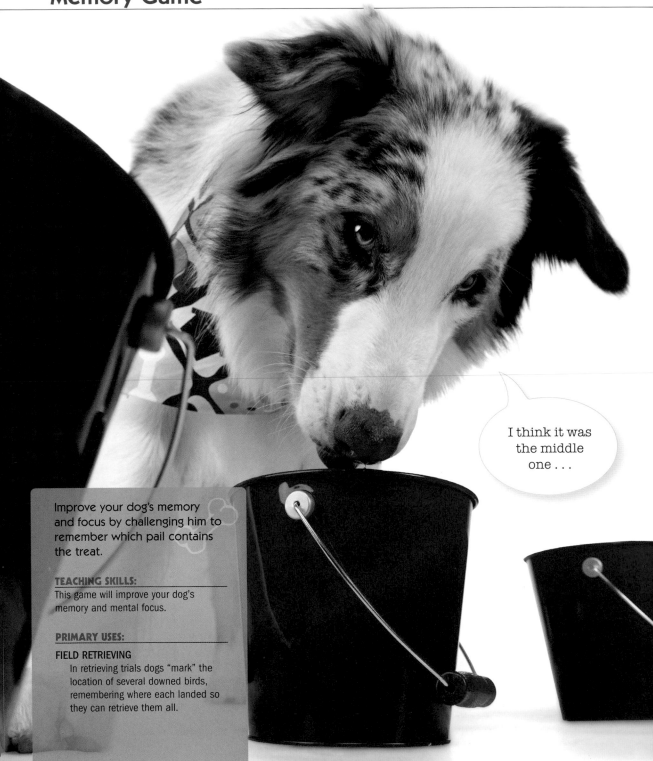

I think it was the middle one . . .

Improve your dog's memory and focus by challenging him to remember which pail contains the treat.

TEACHING SKILLS:

This game will improve your dog's memory and mental focus.

PRIMARY USES:

FIELD RETRIEVING

In retrieving trials dogs "mark" the location of several downed birds, remembering where each landed so they can retrieve them all.

TRY IT:

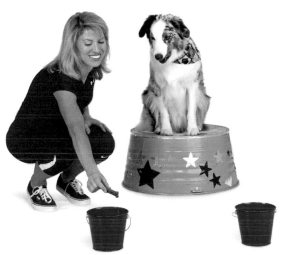

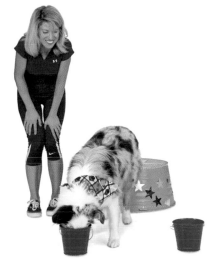

1 Set out two identical pails a few feet apart. Have your dog sit-stay (it is helpful to have him sit on a Pedestal, page 136). Show him as you place a treat into one cup.

2 Go back to him and release him to get the treat. If he goes first to the wrong pail, do not allow him to then check the other pail. Instead, place him back in a sit-stay and start all over.

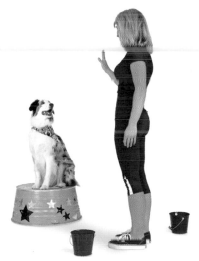

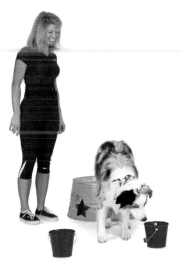

3 Increase the time that your dog must remember. Place a treat in one pail, stand in the center between the pails, and count to five before returning to your dog and releasing him.

4 Try adding a third pail. This will be considerably more difficult for your dog, so go back to having him wait only a minimum amount of time.

TIP:

This game is surprisingly difficult for dogs but provides excellent training for their focus and memory. Even when your dog has mastered the two-pail game, he will find it quite difficult to be successful with three pails.

EQUIPMENT:

Use a pail that is heavy enough that it won't be knocked over, and large enough that your dog can easily reach the treat at the bottom.

BUILD ON IT:

Back-Track Memory Game page 36

Back-Track Memory Game

Improve your dog's extended memory by challenging him to mark the location of a toy and then return to find it.

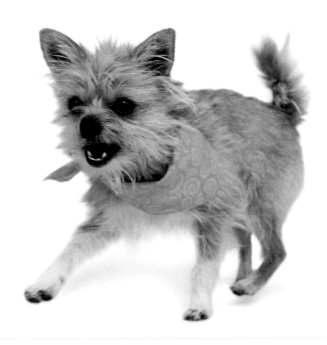

TEACHING SKILLS:

This game improves your dog's memory, mental focus, and scenting ability.

PRIMARY USES:

TRACKING / SEARCH AND RESCUE
In this game your dog will use his scenting ability to help him find the toy or treat. Your dog learns to read the wind and find the scent cone—skills that he will need in the sport of tracking.

TRY IT:

Show your dog his favorite toy (or a food toy) and place it on the ground. Gently take him by the collar and turn him away from the toy. Excitedly say "OK!" and release him to get his reward. Next, place the toy in a new location and walk your dog farther away from the toy.

TIP:

Build distance gradually in order to ensure your dog's success, which will motivate him to try just a little harder with each repetition. Eventually you can back-track a few hundred feet. This game can also be played with multiple dogs—seeing who can find the reward first (end the game if you see signs of aggression).

EQUIPMENT:

Use a target that your dog really wants—for some dogs that may be a toy, and for others it may be food. Food should be placed in a container such as a food-dispensing toy or a bowl so that it will be big enough for your dog to find.

BUILD ON IT:

Treasure Hunt
page 48

Treat under a Blanket

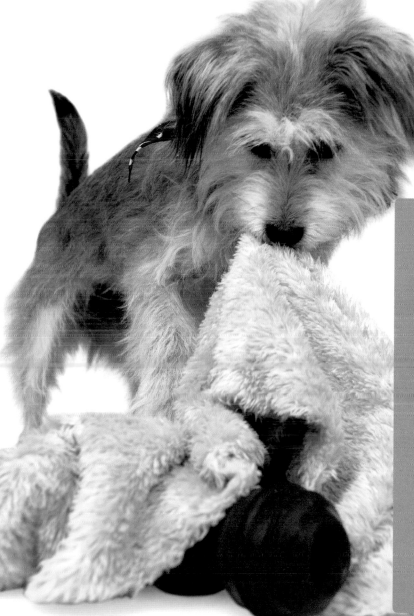

This game challenges your dog to figure out how to get at a toy hidden under a blanket.

TEACHING SKILLS:

This game challenges your dog's mental focus and logic skills.

PRIMARY USES:

SEARCH AND RESCUE
This game is often used to evaluate the drive and persistence of a potential SAR dog. A good SAR dog candidate will struggle repeatedly to get his toy without losing interest.

TRY IT:

Let your dog sniff a food toy to get him interested in it. Place it on the floor and cover it with a blanket. Encourage your dog to "get it!" When he eventually uncovers the toy, let him have the treat as his reward.

TIP:

Some dogs will pursue the toy more vigorously than others. If your dog starts to lose interest, quickly lift up a corner of the blanket so that he can see the toy, and put the blanket back down.

EQUIPMENT:

Use a reward that your dog really likes, such as a peanut-butter-stuffed food toy. The reward should be large enough that your dog can feel it underneath the blanket and have enough smell to keep your dog motivated to find it.

BUILD ON IT:

Tied Up Towel
page 47

Logic Test

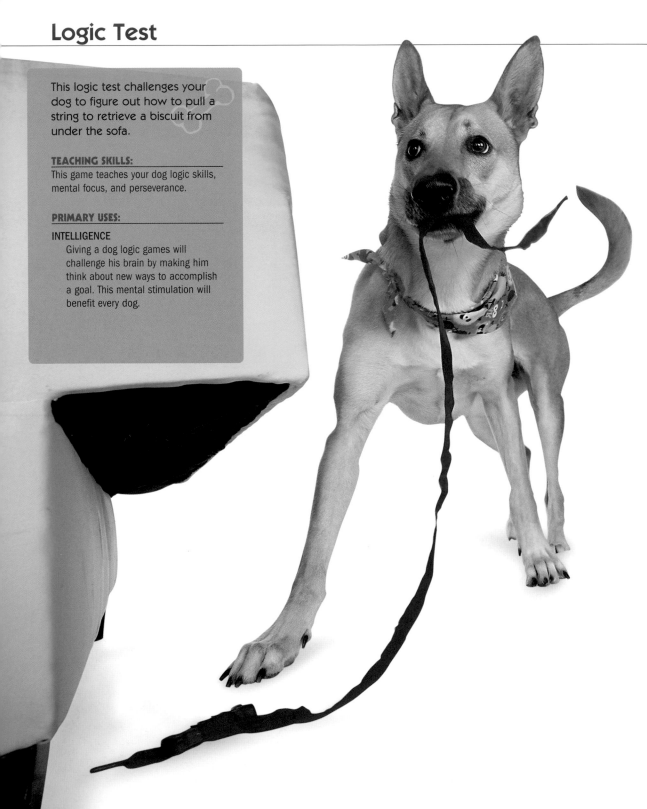

This logic test challenges your dog to figure out how to pull a string to retrieve a biscuit from under the sofa.

TEACHING SKILLS:
This game teaches your dog logic skills, mental focus, and perseverance.

PRIMARY USES:

INTELLIGENCE
Giving a dog logic games will challenge his brain by making him think about new ways to accomplish a goal. This mental stimulation will benefit every dog.

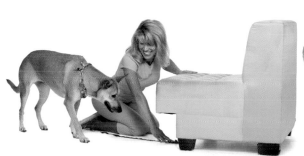

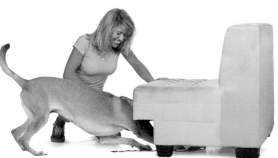

1 Tie a thick string around a dog biscuit. Let your dog watch as you push the biscuit about 18 inches (45 cm) under the sofa. The string should be visible on the floor.

2 Your dog will try various tactics to get the biscuit, such as sticking his nose under the sofa and pawing under the sofa.

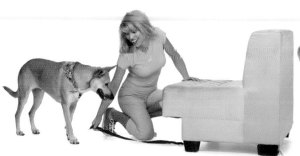

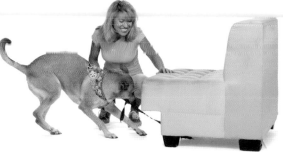

3 After a minute, let your dog watch as you pull the string to reveal the biscuit. Do not let your dog have the biscuit. Repeat this a second time. Again, do not let your dog have the biscuit.

4 On the third repetition, wait for your dog figure out how to pull the string himself. You may have to point at the string or wiggle it to help him get the idea.

TIP:	EQUIPMENT:	BUILD ON IT:
This fun, ten-minute game is perfect for rainy days. It may take your dog a few tries to figure out how to pull the string, but once he does, he will enjoy pulling biscuits out from all sorts of places.	Use a crunchy biscuit that will crumble when your dog bites it, so that he will not accidentally swallow the string. Watch closely in any case and do not allow your dog to eat the string.	Fishing with a Rope *page 40*

Fishing with a Rope

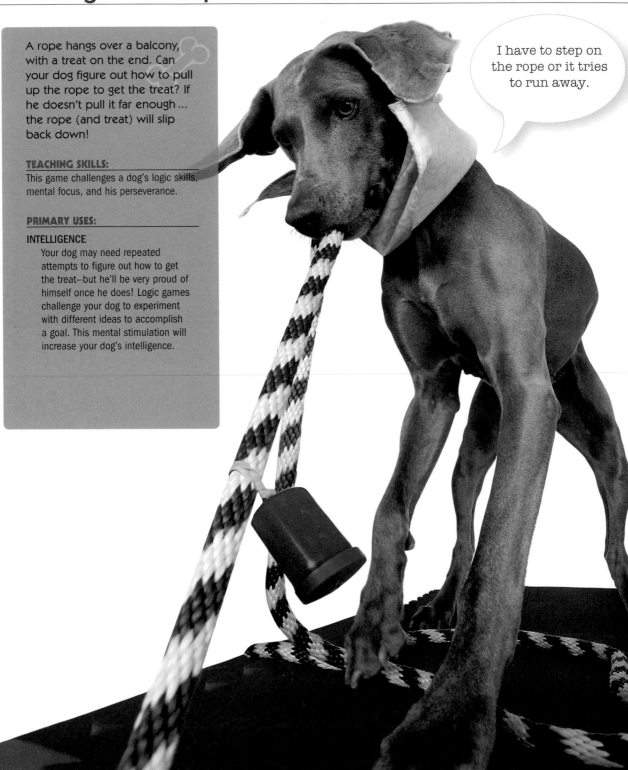

A rope hangs over a balcony, with a treat on the end. Can your dog figure out how to pull up the rope to get the treat? If he doesn't pull it far enough ... the rope (and treat) will slip back down!

TEACHING SKILLS:
This game challenges a dog's logic skills, mental focus, and his perseverance.

PRIMARY USES:

INTELLIGENCE
Your dog may need repeated attempts to figure out how to get the treat—but he'll be very proud of himself once he does! Logic games challenge your dog to experiment with different ideas to accomplish a goal. This mental stimulation will increase your dog's intelligence.

I have to step on the rope or it tries to run away.

TRY IT:

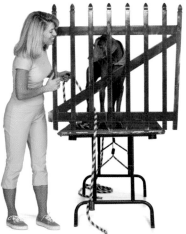

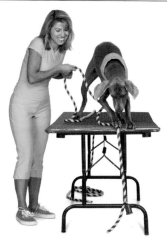

1 This game is easiest taught with your dog behind a railing, such as you might find on a staircase or balcony. Attach a treat (in a container) to the end of the rope. Show your dog the treat and then hang the rope 2 feet (61 cm) over the edge.

2 Your dog may bite or scratch at the rope. Reward each of his attempts by pulling the rope a few inches toward him.

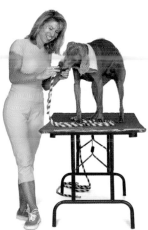

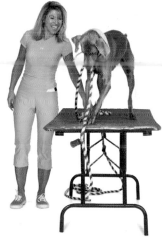

3 Once he manages to pull the treat container up, open it and let him take the treat. It is important to let him have the reward from the container and not a different treat from your pocket.

4 Once your dog gets the hang of it, let him pull up the rope all by himself. Eventually your dog will bite the rope and back up, pulling up the treat.

TIP:

Each dog will go through a unique set of trial-and-error attempts until he figures out how to pull up the treat. Don't worry if your dog is not getting it at first . . . allow him time to figure it out on his own.

EQUIPMENT:

Use a thick rope of about ¾-inch (2 cm) diameter. A waste-pickup-bag cylinder works well as a food container to attach to the rope. Try this game at the top of a staircase, with the rope hanging between the rails of the banister. Your dog may scratch at the rope, so you may wish to protect your stairs with a doormat.

BUILD ON IT:

Logic Test
page 38

Fishing with a Rope   **41**

Focus on Trainer

When you have your dog's eyes, you have his attention. This game teaches your dog to focus on your eyes.

TEACHING SKILLS:

This game teaches mental focus and self-control.

PRIMARY USES:

FOUNDATION SKILL

Teaching your dog to give you attention is the basis for all training. Focus exercises are a foundation skill practiced in almost every dog sport.

CONFIDENCE

Shy dogs may be reluctant to look into your eyes, possibly because they wish to avoid confrontation. This exercise will be especially helpful for shy dogs.

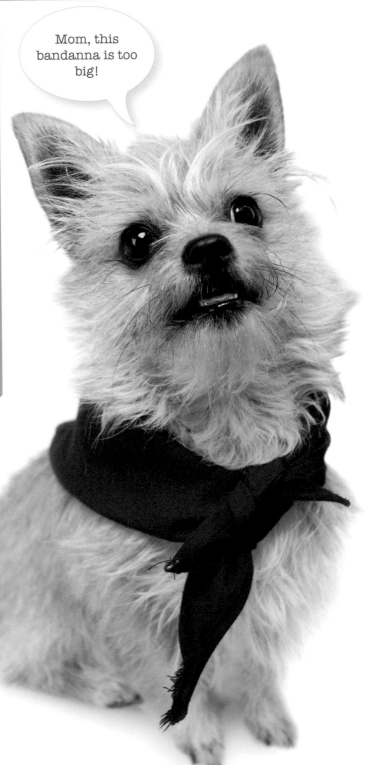

Mom, this bandanna is too big!

TRY IT:

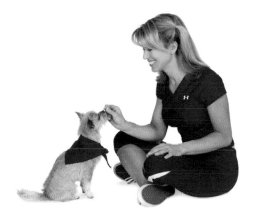

1 Kneel down to your dog's height. Hold a treat at your dog's eye level.

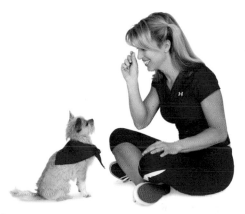

2 Slowly bring the treat back toward your eyes. In a calm, drawn-out voice say, "Focus . . . Focus . . ."

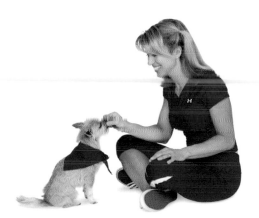

3 Once your dog holds eye contact for a second or two, say, "Good!" and give him the treat. You want your dog to be successful, so try to reward him before he loses interest and looks away.

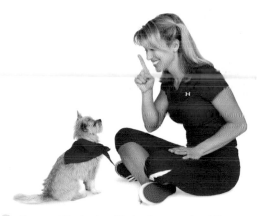

4 Phase out the treat and instead use a pointed finger between your eyes and the word "focus" as your cue. When your dog holds his stare, say "good!" and give him a treat. As he improves, you can require longer stares before you reward.

TIP:

Make a habit of requiring a moment of calm attention before routine rewards, such as at the front door before a walk, or at the food dish before chow time. As soon as your dog holds eye contact for a second or two, give him his reward. This will teach your dog self-control, and that calm, attentive behavior is rewarded.

EQUIPMENT:

Remove your sunglasses. It may help to kneel down so that your dog can more easily look into your eyes.

BUILD ON IT:

Balance & Catch
page 44

Follow Pointed Finger
page 130

Balance & Catch

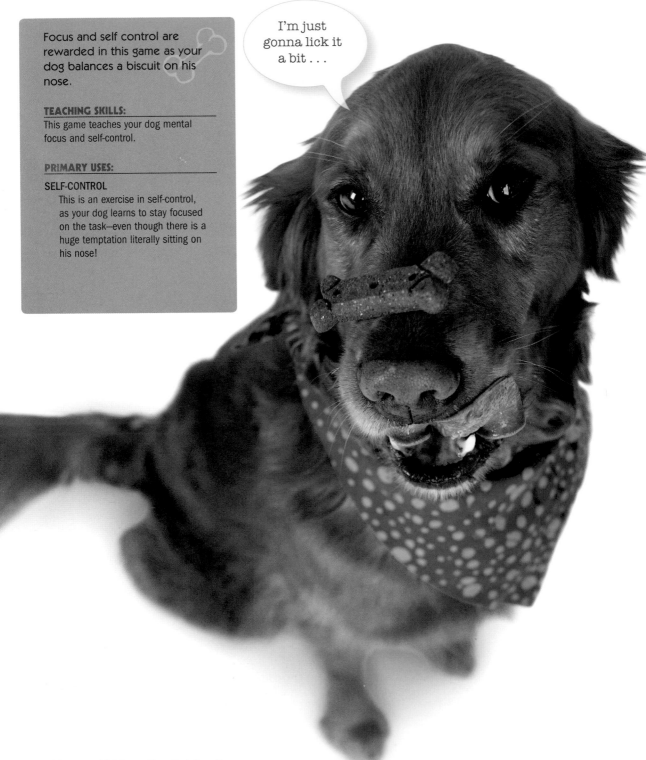

Focus and self control are rewarded in this game as your dog balances a biscuit on his nose.

TEACHING SKILLS:

This game teaches your dog mental focus and self-control.

PRIMARY USES:

SELF-CONTROL
This is an exercise in self-control, as your dog learns to stay focused on the task—even though there is a huge temptation literally sitting on his nose!

I'm just gonna lick it a bit . . .

TRY IT:

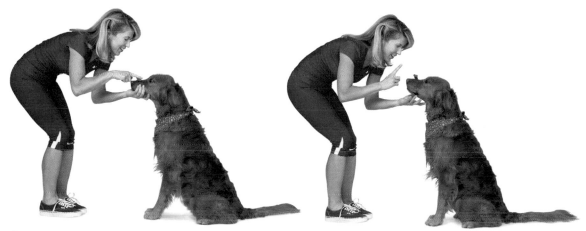

1 Start with your dog in a sit. Gently hold his muzzle parallel to the floor and balance a treat on the bridge of his nose. In a low voice, coach him to "waaaaaait . . . "

2 Use a pointed finger to focus his attention. Slowly release his muzzle.

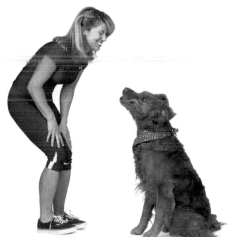

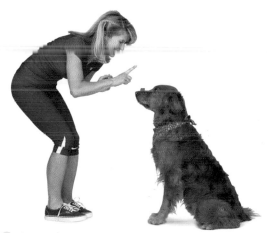

3 After a second of your dog holding this position, say, "Catch!" as the release word.

4 As your dog improves, see if he can hold this position longer. Or try having him balance different objects on his nose. Continue to use your pointed finger to focus his attention.

TIP:

The purpose of this game is to improve your dog's focus and self-control. It is not important that he be able to catch the treat which he has flipped from his nose (although some dogs can!)

EQUIPMENT:

Pug-nosed breeds will have a harder time balancing a treat. Make it easier for your dog by using a flexible treat such as a wet noodle or strip of deli meat.

BUILD ON IT:

Soap
Bubbles
page 158

Muffin Tin

All dogs love this game! Hide treats in a muffin tin, cover the cups with tennis balls, and watch your dog sniff them out.

TEACHING SKILLS:

This game improves your dog's scenting ability, logic skills, and mental focus.

PRIMARY USES:

NOSE WORK

In this introduction to nose work, your dog learns that using his nose produces rewards.

TRY IT:

Place three or four strongly scented treats in a muffin tin, each in its own compartment. Place a ball on top of each opening in the tray, concealing the treats underneath. Put the tin on the floor and let your dog figure out how to get the treats.

We've done this a thousand times. Didn't you get the picture yet?

TIP:

With a very enthusiastic dog, you might need to hold the muffin tin in place. With a reluctant dog, put treats in every cup and put balls over only half of the cups.

EQUIPMENT:

Use an ordinary muffin tin and a dozen tennis balls.

BUILD ON IT:

Nose Work Box Search
page 50

Tied-Up Towel

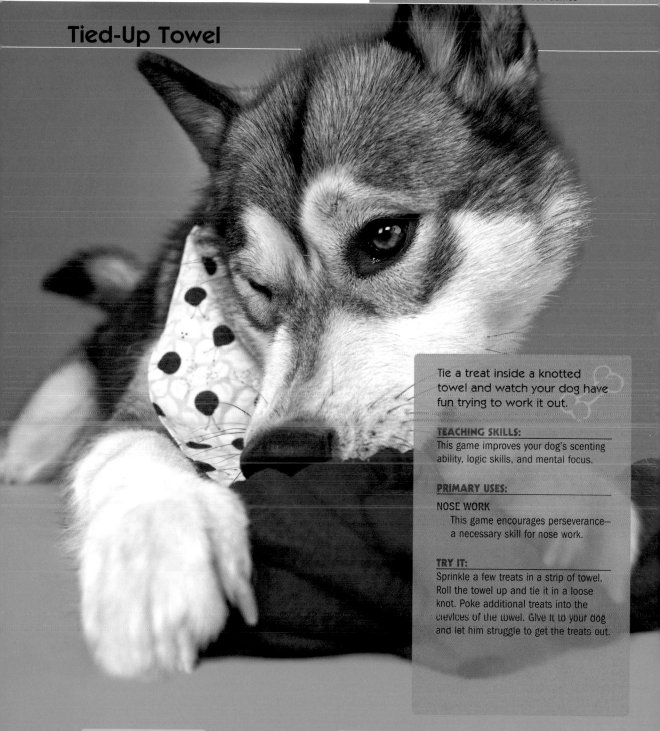

Tie a treat inside a knotted towel and watch your dog have fun trying to work it out.

TEACHING SKILLS:

This game improves your dog's scenting ability, logic skills, and mental focus.

PRIMARY USES:

NOSE WORK

This game encourages perseverance—a necessary skill for nose work.

TRY IT:

Sprinkle a few treats in a strip of towel. Roll the towel up and tie it in a loose knot. Poke additional treats into the crevices of the towel. Give it to your dog and let him struggle to get the treats out.

TIP:

Supervise your dog to make sure he does not try to eat the towel. For less tenacious dogs, simply roll up the towel with the treats and do not tie it in a knot.

EQUIPMENT:

Use a thin dish towel, or cut an old towel into strips to make it less bulky.

BUILD ON IT:

Treat under a Blanket
page 37

Treasure Hunt

Hide some treats or toys around the house and have your dog go on a treasure hunt to find them.

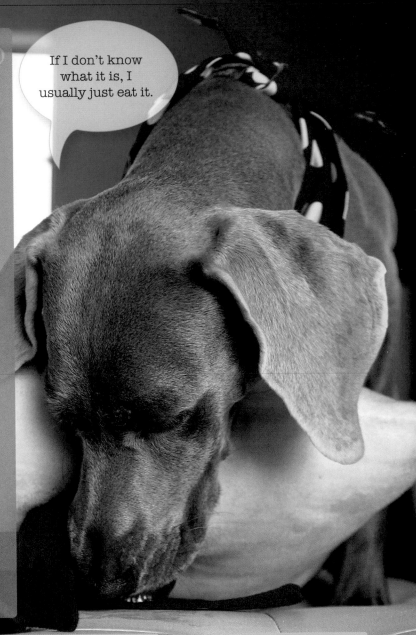

If I don't know what it is, I usually just eat it.

TEACHING SKILLS:

This fun game improves your dog's scenting ability, mental focus, and independent hunting skills.

PRIMARY USES:

NOSE WORK

This game teaches your dog to search for the hidden scent in a variety of places—high, low, under furniture, and in unusual places. This game prepares him for the "building search" exercise in nose work.

SEARCH AND RESCUE

SAR dogs must have the mental focus and persistence to continue searching for their goal for long periods of time. This game provides a rewarding way to develop those skills in your dog.

TRY IT:

Hide a few treats in plain view. Point to them and encourage your dog to "find it!" Make it more challenging by hiding treats at different elevations, under the sofa, in several rooms, and in unusual places. Your dog will have fun running around the house sniffing them out!

TIP:

If your dog seems confused, encourage him by pointing toward the treat. When you increase the difficulty, make sure your dog is still having good success, as you don't want him to become frustrated and give up.

EQUIPMENT:

If your dog really loves a specific toy, use that for the hidden treasure. Otherwise use small treats such as kibble, goldfish crackers, popcorn, or Cheerios cereal. For a low-calorie treat use raw fruits and vegetables (such as carrots, green beans, potatoes, broccoli, and apples.)

BUILD ON IT:

Muffin Tin
page 46

Which Hand Holds the Treat?

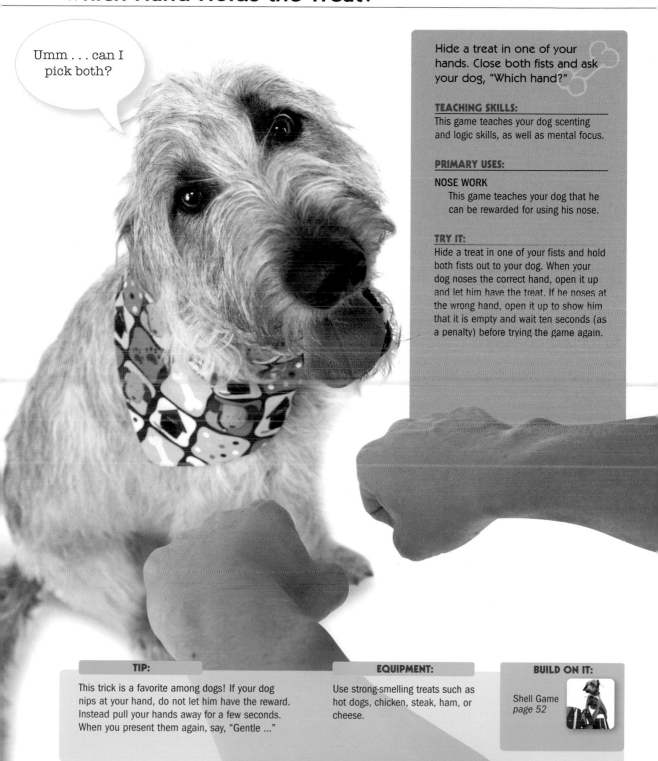

Umm . . . can I pick both?

Hide a treat in one of your hands. Close both fists and ask your dog, "Which hand?"

TEACHING SKILLS:

This game teaches your dog scenting and logic skills, as well as mental focus.

PRIMARY USES:

NOSE WORK

This game teaches your dog that he can be rewarded for using his nose.

TRY IT:

Hide a treat in one of your fists and hold both fists out to your dog. When your dog noses the correct hand, open it up and let him have the treat. If he noses at the wrong hand, open it up to show him that it is empty and wait ten seconds (as a penalty) before trying the game again.

TIP:

This trick is a favorite among dogs! If your dog nips at your hand, do not let him have the reward. Instead pull your hands away for a few seconds. When you present them again, say, "Gentle ..."

EQUIPMENT:

Use strong-smelling treats such as hot dogs, chicken, steak, ham, or cheese.

BUILD ON IT:

Shell Game
page 52

Nose Work Box Search

A dog needs confidence to work independently. In this nose-work game, the handler takes a backseat as the dog sniffs boxes to find the one containing a target scent.

TEACHING SKILLS:

This exercise tests a dog's scenting ability, mental focus, and willingness to hunt independently.

PRIMARY USES:

NOSE WORK

This box search game is one of the basic tests in the sport of nose work.

DETECTION DOG

The sport of nose work is derived from the work performed by scent detection dogs (such as bomb-sniffing or drug-sniffing dogs). They also must search multiple containers for a target scent.

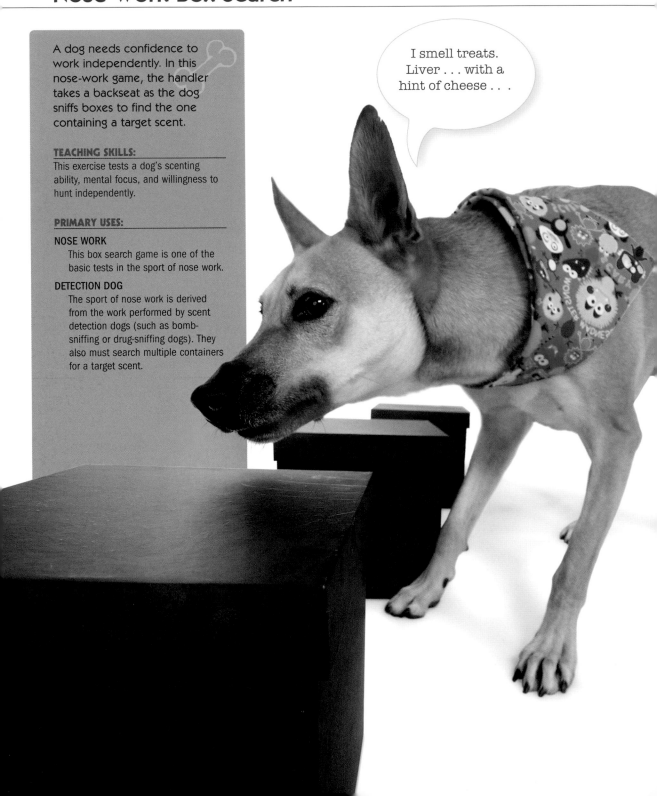

I smell treats. Liver . . . with a hint of cheese . . .

TRY IT:

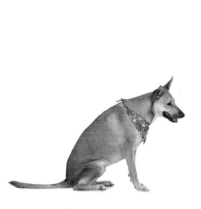

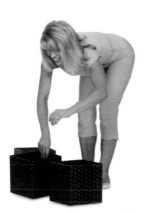

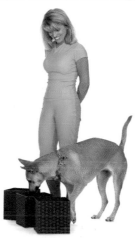

1 Set out three to six open boxes. Put some strong-smelling treats in a pouch or ventilated container (so your dog can't eat them). Hide the treat container in one of the boxes and mix them up so your dog doesn't know which box has the "hide."

2 Release your dog to search the boxes. Don't say anything while your dog searches, as it will distract him. If your dog needs encouragement, nonchalantly investigate the boxes yourself.

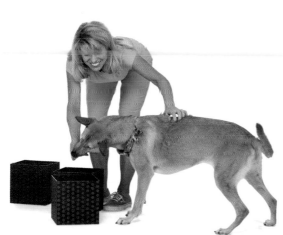

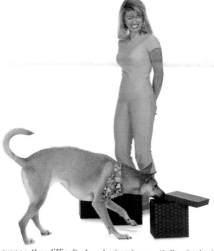

3 As soon your dog shows any interest in the correct box, enthusiastically praise him and give him a treat. (Always give the treat next to the correct box.)

4 Increase the difficulty by closing (or partially closing) the boxes. Punch holes in the boxes for ventilation, so your dog can smell the treats inside.

TIP:

Nose work is a team sport; your dog finds the target scent, and you read his body language to know when he has found it. Watch your dog and learn to pick up on subtle body and breathing changes that indicate that he is on the trail of his target. Keep your sessions short and fun.

EQUIPMENT:

A variety of containers can work for this game: cardboard boxes, plastic food storage containers with holes punched in them, or upturned flower pots. It is helpful, but not imperative, for the containers to be identical.

BUILD ON IT:

Shell Game
page 52

Shell Game

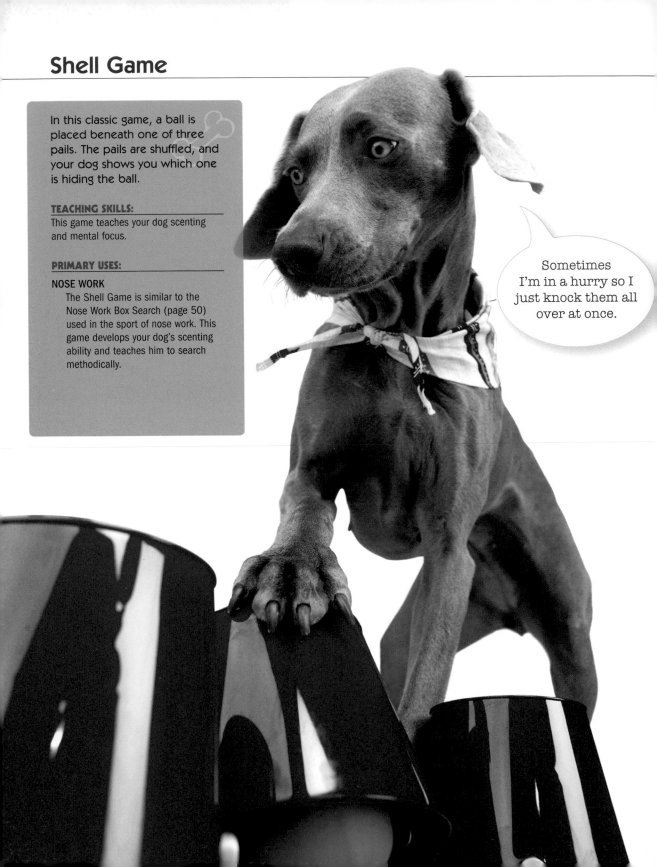

In this classic game, a ball is placed beneath one of three pails. The pails are shuffled, and your dog shows you which one is hiding the ball.

TEACHING SKILLS:

This game teaches your dog scenting and mental focus.

PRIMARY USES:

NOSE WORK

The Shell Game is similar to the Nose Work Box Search (page 50) used in the sport of nose work. This game develops your dog's scenting ability and teaches him to search methodically.

Sometimes I'm in a hurry so I just knock them all over at once.

TRY IT:

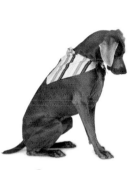
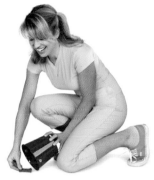
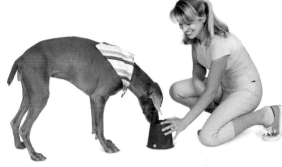

1. Start with just one pail. Rub the inside with a treat, or tape a treat to the inside against the scent hole. Show your dog as you place a treat on the floor and cover it with the pail.

2. Encourage your dog to "find it!" When he noses or paws the pail, say, "Good!" and lift the pail, allowing him to get the treat.

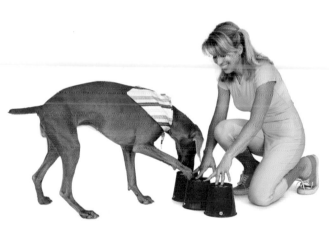
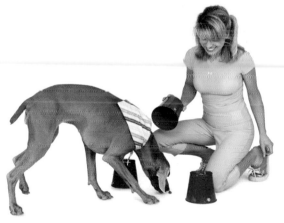

3. Add two more pails. You may have to hold them down so that your dog doesn't knock them over. If he indicates an incorrect pail, do not lift it, but encourage him to "keep looking."

4. When your dog shows significant interest in the correct pail, say, "Good!" and lift it.

TIP:

This game can be confusing for your dog at first, so be gentle and avoid saying "no." If your dog loses interest, quickly lift the pail to reveal the treat, and replace the pail. Always end this game on a successful attempt to keep your dog motivated and looking forward to the next time!

EQUIPMENT:

Use three identical pails which have a hole in their base to allow your dog to smell the contents. Heavy clay flower pots work well, as they have a hole in their base and won't overturn easily.

BUILD ON IT:

Scent Discrimination
page 54

Scent Discrimination

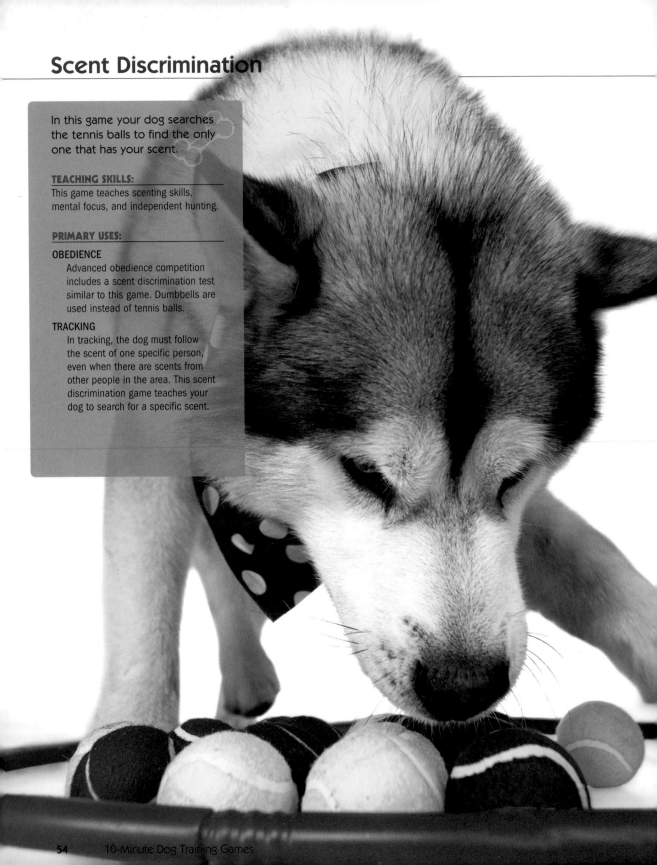

In this game your dog searches the tennis balls to find the only one that has your scent.

TEACHING SKILLS:
This game teaches scenting skills, mental focus, and independent hunting.

PRIMARY USES:

OBEDIENCE
Advanced obedience competition includes a scent discrimination test similar to this game. Dumbbells are used instead of tennis balls.

TRACKING
In tracking, the dog must follow the scent of one specific person, even when there are scents from other people in the area. This scent discrimination game teaches your dog to search for a specific scent.

TRY IT:

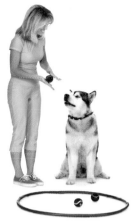

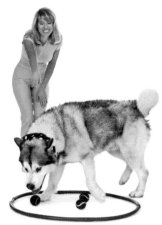

1 Start by teaching your dog to Fetch (page 144). Set out three unscented balls. Scent one by rubbing it in your palms, and also with some of your treats. (Remember to mark the balls so you can tell which is the scented one!)

2 Point to the balls and instruct your dog to, "Find mine, fetch!" If your dog starts to fetch a wrong ball, keep pointing to and looking at the other balls, and say encouragingly, "Find mine!"

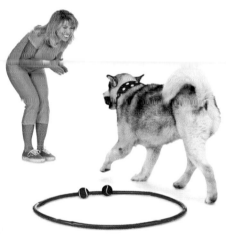

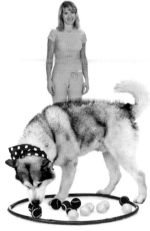

3 As soon as your dog puts his mouth on the correct ball, encourage him back to you, saying, "Good boy, bring it here." Give him a treat when he brings the correct ball.

4 Fairly soon, increase the number of balls in the set. Once your dog starts to understand the goal, it will be helpful for you to keep quiet, as this will give him the confidence to work independently.

TIP:

Some dogs get the hang of this game in ten minutes. All dogs, however, will go through periods of doubt, where they regress. Know that this is part of the learning process and do not become frustrated and do not reprimand your dog for choosing incorrectly. Instead, just encourage him to go back and find the correct ball.

EQUIPMENT:

The tennis balls must be scent-free, so handle them with tongs and air them out for a day between uses. Use a hoop to confine them so that they don't roll around the room.

BUILD ON IT:

Tracking
page 58

Rapporthund
page 60

Hide & Seek

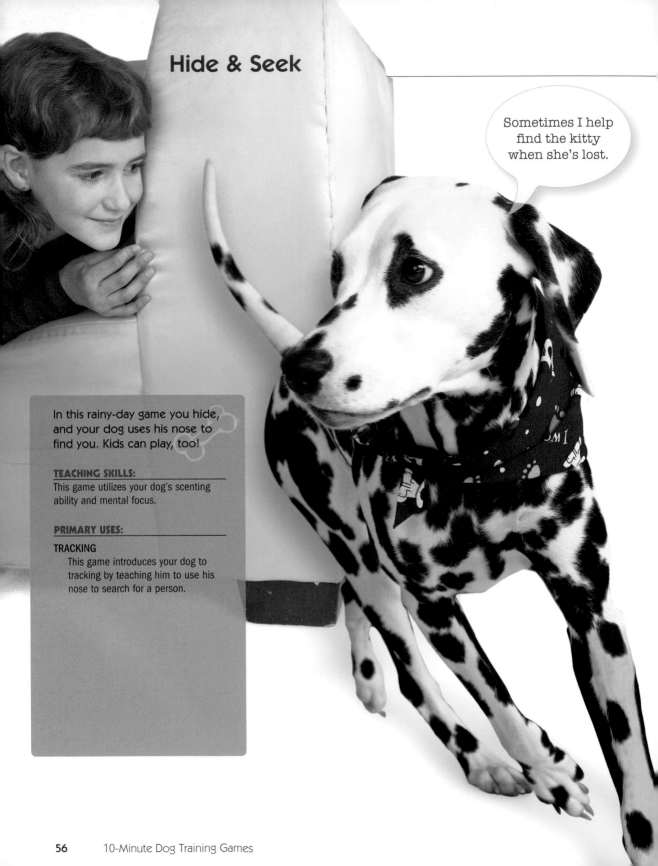

Sometimes I help find the kitty when she's lost.

In this rainy-day game you hide, and your dog uses his nose to find you. Kids can play, too!

TEACHING SKILLS:
This game utilizes your dog's scenting ability and mental focus.

PRIMARY USES:

TRACKING
This game introduces your dog to tracking by teaching him to use his nose to search for a person.

TRY IT:

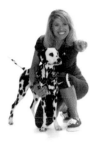

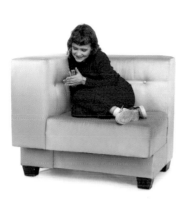

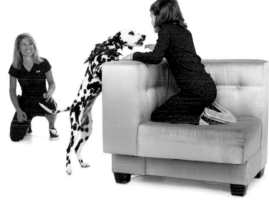

1 Your dog will be most motivated to search for people he is bonded with, such as family members. Hold your dog while the other person hides nearby; perhaps behind a piece of furniture.

2 Tell your dog to "find [person's name]!" The hiding person can help by calling to the dog. When your dog reaches them, the person gives a treat to your dog.

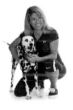

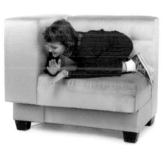

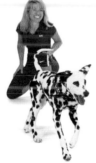

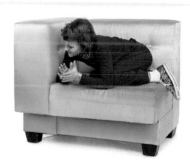

3 Gradually use more difficult hiding spots, such as behind an open door, in the chowor, or in a partially open closet. Always give a treat or an enthusiastic play session as a reward for your dog finding his target.

4 Your dog will learn to use his nose to scent for the person. He will even be able to scent the path that the person walked to their hiding place (you can try to fool your dog by walking into multiple rooms before hiding!).

TIP:

Dogs love this game! When the dog is busy getting his reward from one person, the other person can then hide, and you can play again with the roles reversed.

BUILD ON IT:

Rapporthund
page 60

Tracking

Your dog has an amazing nose. Teach him to use it to follow a person's trail.

TEACHING SKILLS:

Tracking teaches scenting, mental focus, and independent hunting skills.

PRIMARY USES:

TRACKING

Tracking is its own sport, and it is also a component of Schutzhund competition. In competition a tracklayer walks across a field, dropping several items along the way. The dog must find the items (which he indicates by lying down), and must find the person or item at the end of the track.

SEARCH & RESCUE

SAR dogs must be able to follow a scent trail 1 mile (1.6 km) in distance.

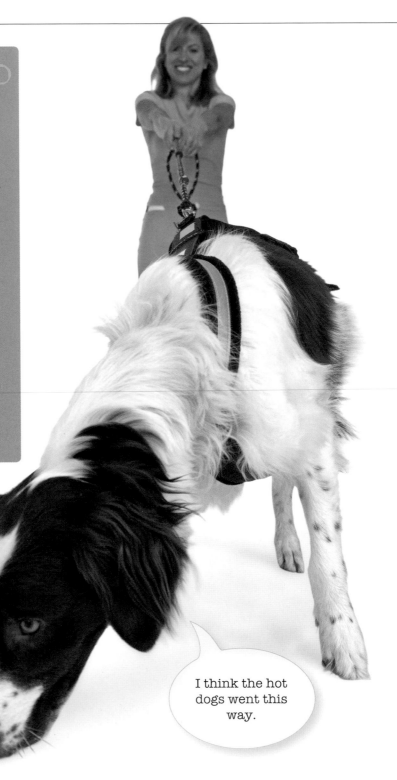

I think the hot dogs went this way.

TRY IT:

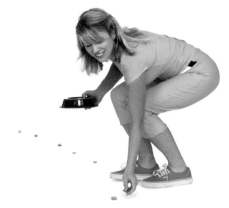

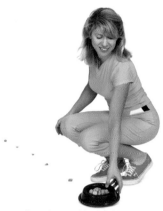

1 Have your dog wait in the car while you walk a 50-meter (164 feet) straight line, scuffing your feet along the way. As you walk, drop strong smelling treats every few steps.

2 Place a big reward, such as a big dog biscuit or a favorite toy, at the end of the trail.

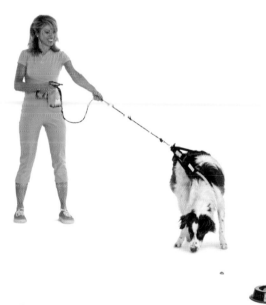

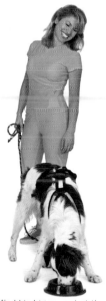

3 Start your dog at the beginning of the trail and allow him to pull you along the trail as he gobbles up the treats.

4 Let your dog find his big reward at the end!

TIP:

If your dog veers off track, be aware that the scent may be traveling on the breeze, and he may still be following the trail. As your dog improves, space the treats farther apart and put gradual bends in your track.

EQUIPMENT:

Outfit your dog in a harness and 12-foot (3.7 m) lead. Lay your track in moist grass, as it holds more scent and will be easier for your dog to follow. Use garden flags to remind you of the path you traveled.

BUILD ON IT:

Back-Track Memory Game
page 36

Rapporthund
page 60

Rapporthund

In this game your dog carries a top-secret message back and forth between two people, just like traditional war dogs did.

TEACHING SKILLS:

This useful game teaches your dog scenting skills, confidence, independent hunting, and mental focus.

PRIMARY USES:

MESSENGER DOG COMPETITION
Patterned after traditional war dog duties, the sport of Rapporthund (or messenger dog) entails a dog carrying a message on his collar back and forth between two people. Competitions are timed, with the fastest dog being the winner.

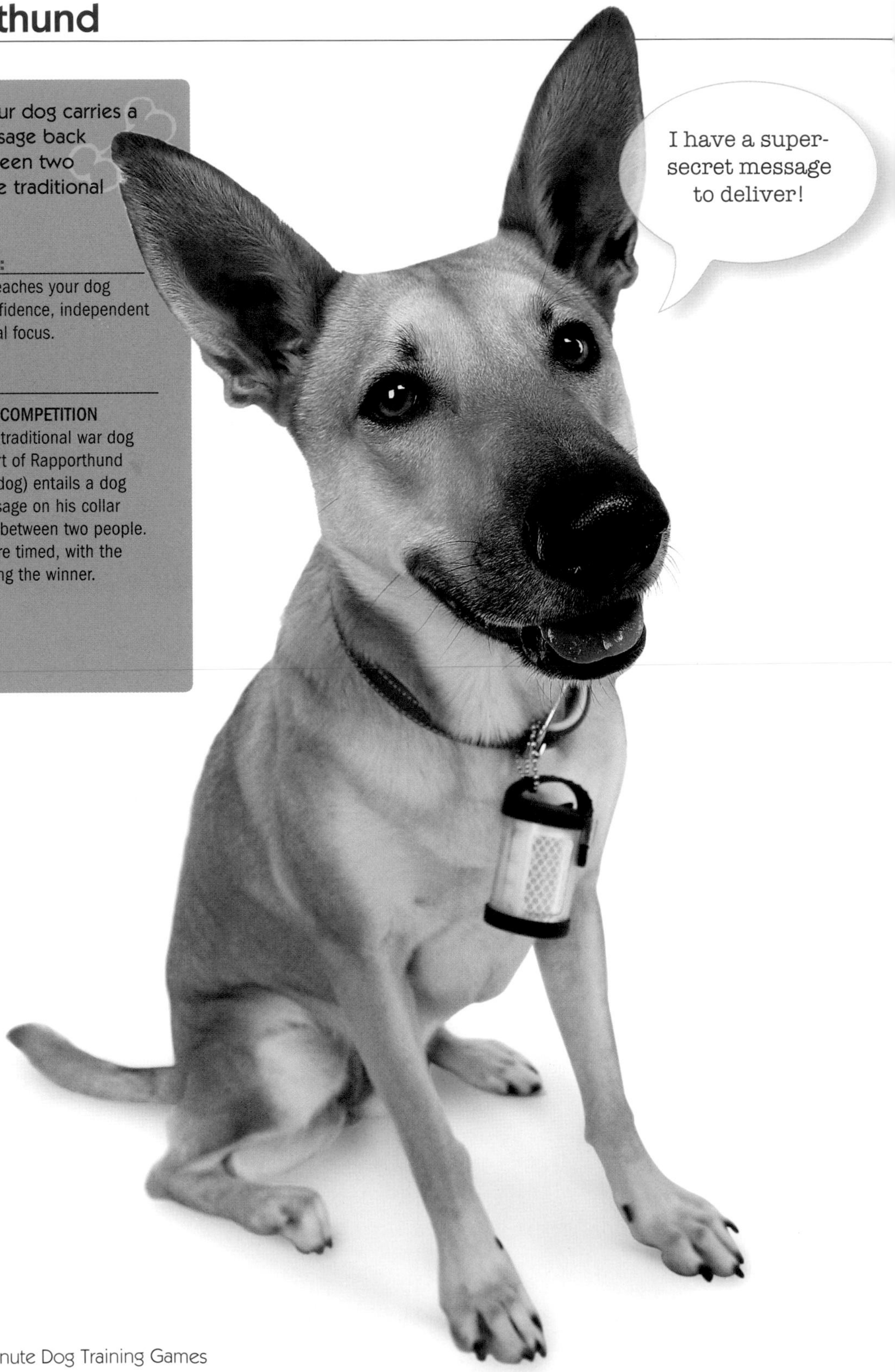

I have a super-secret message to deliver!

TRY IT:

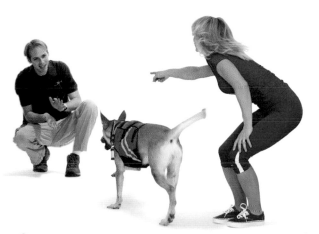

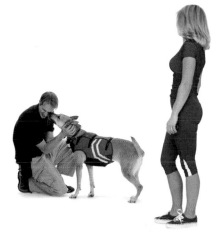

1 Play this game with two people that your dog is bonded with, such as family members. Start in a boring environment, such as your home or yard. Separate and send the dog to the other person, saying, "Find [person's name]!"

2 As the dog approaches him, the recipient should clap and encourage the dog. When the dog arrives, the recipient gives the dog enthusiastic praise and a handful of yummy treats.

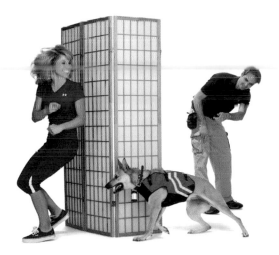

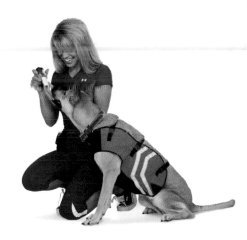

3 Now make it more difficult. Have the other person hold your dog while you run away and disappear around a corner. Can your dog still find you?

4 After you've sent your dog, take that opportunity to hide yourself in a new spot. Keep the game going, sending your dog back and forth between people.

TIP:

As your distance increases, your dog will rely more upon his scenting ability to find you and will track the path you walked. This exercise can come in handy if you ever lose your spouse or child!

EQUIPMENT:

No piece of equipment is absolutely necessary for this game; however, some items that may be helpful are a blaze-orange dog vest, a collar message canister, a GPS tracking collar, and cellphones or radios.

BUILD ON IT:

Back-Track Memory Game
page 36

Massage

Massage provides physical benefits to your dog and also conditions him to go into a relaxation mode.

TEACHING SKILLS:

Massage promotes relaxation, bonding, and mental focus.

PRIMARY USES:

REHABILITATION

Massage loosens tight muscles and relieves pain from arthritis, hip dysplasia, and stiffness associated with old age.

BONDING

Massage reduces stress and helps your dog to feel comfortable with people touching him (which will help with nail trimming and grooming).

PERFORMANCE SPORTS

Canine athletes benefit from a cooldown massage, which loosens them physically and mentally.

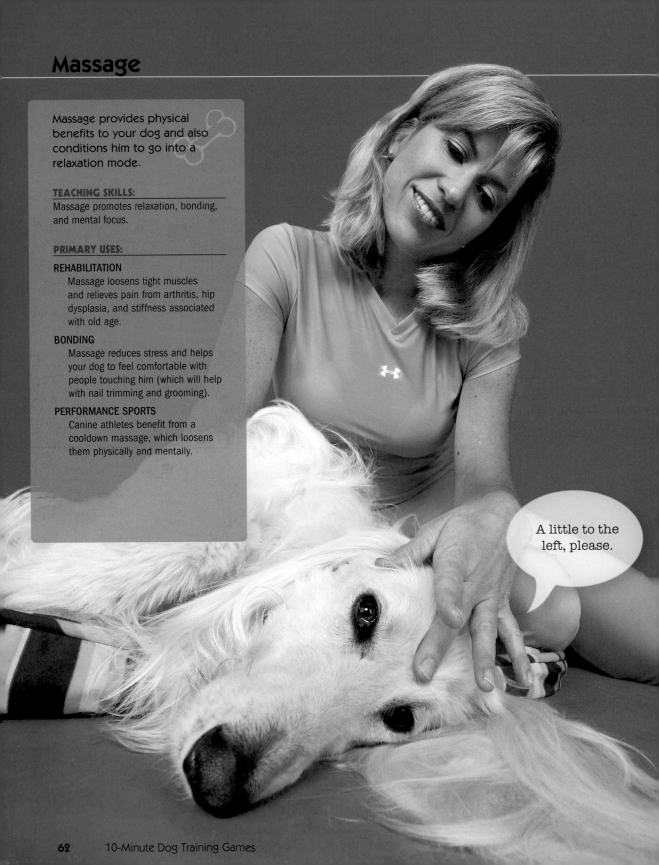

A little to the left, please.

TRY IT:

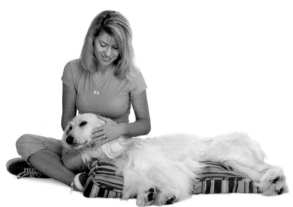

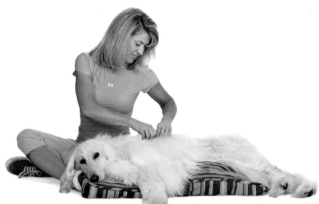

1 Start by loosening your dog's muscles. Use a flat hand to stroke softly from head to tail. Scratch behind the ears; rub along the cheeks and under the chin, over the nose, and between the eyes.

2 Use light pressure and small, circular strokes on muscular areas. Use three fingers on each side of the leg, rubbing softly in opposite directions. When you move to the neck, shoulders, and chest, gently pinch small folds of loose skin.

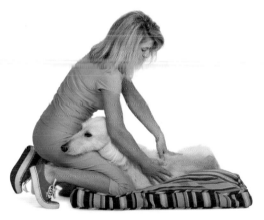

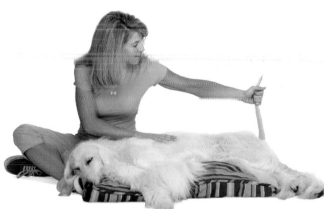

3 Walk your thumb and index finger down the length of the spine—not directly on the spine, but rather along the long muscles on either side. Use your clawed hand to gently vibrate your dog's skin all over his body. If your dog is comfortable with it, give his paws a prolonged and gentle squeeze.

4 Use both hands to rock your dog's body in the same way you'd rock a baby. Squeeze his tail (but don't pull) gently and firmly, from base to tip. End with those long, slow strokes again. If all goes well, you may find you've put your dog to sleep by the end of the ten-minute session.

TIP:	EQUIPMENT:	BUILD ON IT:
Keep your massage light and gentle. Serious, deep massage should only be done by a trained practitioner. Avoid pressing on your dog's stomach.	Have your dog lie on a soft, firm surface.	Doga page 64

Doga

Doga combines meditation, gentle stretching, and relaxation for dogs and their owners. Use this time to bond with your dog.

TEACHING SKILLS:
Doga promotes relaxation, bonding, and mental focus.

PRIMARY USES:

DOGA
Doga classes encourage owners to integrate their dogs into their yoga sessions to promote relaxation and bonding for both owner and dog.

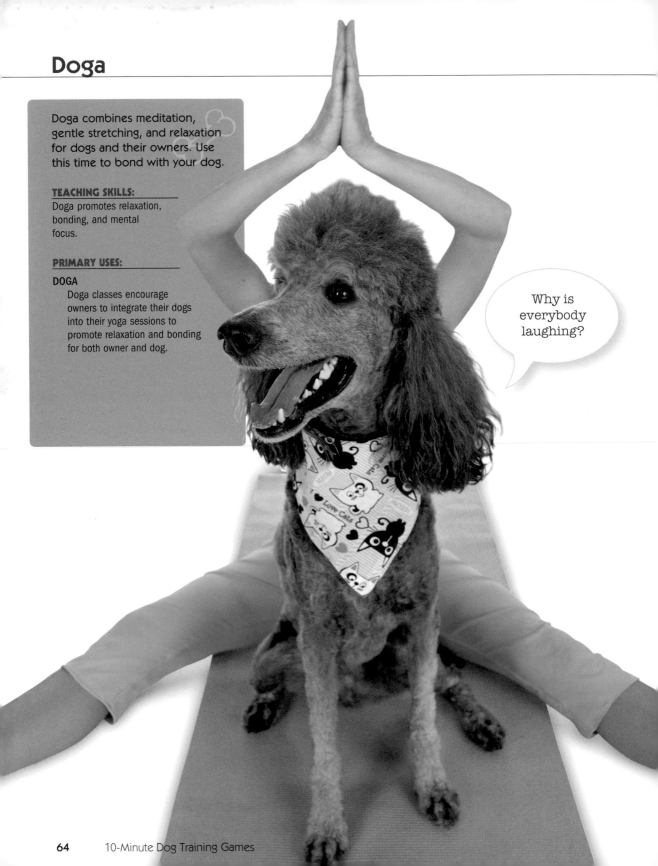

Why is everybody laughing?

TRY IT:

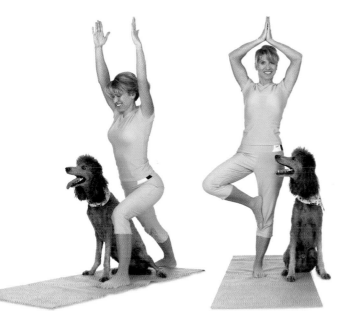

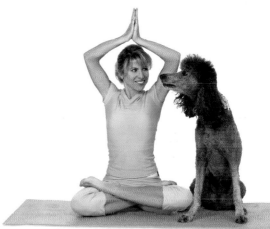

1 As you perform your doga moves, think about joining your intentions with your dog's. It is not to use treats during doga, as treats would energize rather than relax your dog.

2 Connect the energy of your minds. Build the association between the yoga mat and calmness. Introduce the mat to your dog and just sit quietly together.

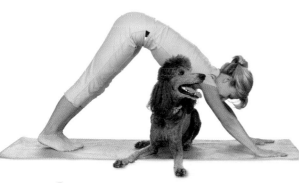

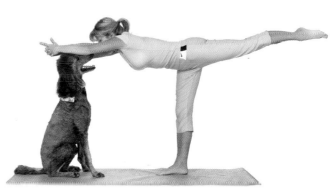

3 Give and receive healing energy. Because dogs are pack animals, they are a natural match for doga's emphasis on union and connection with other beings.

4 Focus on the love between you and your dog. Doga teaches us to be present with our dogs, while encouraging us to be more present and loving in all aspects of our lives.

Cavalettis

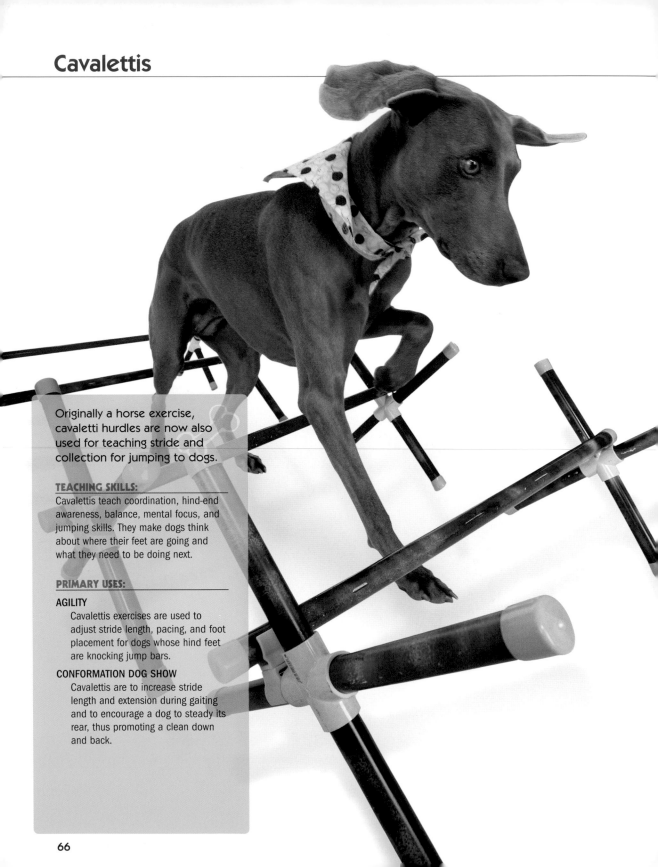

Originally a horse exercise, cavaletti hurdles are now also used for teaching stride and collection for jumping to dogs.

TEACHING SKILLS:
Cavalettis teach coordination, hind-end awareness, balance, mental focus, and jumping skills. They make dogs think about where their feet are going and what they need to be doing next.

PRIMARY USES:

AGILITY
Cavalettis exercises are used to adjust stride length, pacing, and foot placement for dogs whose hind feet are knocking jump bars.

CONFORMATION DOG SHOW
Cavalettis are to increase stride length and extension during gaiting and to encourage a dog to steady its rear, thus promoting a clean down and back.

TRY IT:

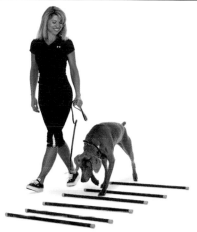

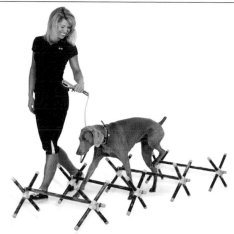

1 Teach foot placement. Lay eight parallel bars at varying distances apart and walk your dog on lead through them. Your dog will probably avoid the bars with his front feet but may step on them with his rear feet. Walk the bars in both directions and with your dog on both sides of you. Do this five to ten times per session for five days.

2 Teach rhythm/cadence. Next, raise the bars and space them equally apart (see "Equipment"). Take your dog through at a slow trot. You don't want him jumping over the bars, but rather stepping (or reaching) over them. As he improves, try different speeds.

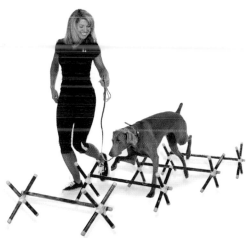

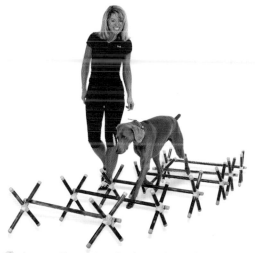

3 Teach maximum stride length. Space the bars at a distance of one and a half times your dog's height at his withers. Take your dog through at a fast trot.

4 Increase the number of poles to sixteen. Gait your dog through the cavalettis ten to fifteen times once or twice a day.

TIP:	EQUIPMENT:	BUILD ON IT:

Avoid using treats as they will distract your dog from thinking about his foot placement.

The bar height should be one-half the height of the dog's hock (rear ankle). Vary the height of the bars slightly so that your dog has to pay attention to each bar. The distance between the bars should be equal to the height of your dog's withers (shoulders).

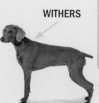

WITHERS

← **HOCK**

Ladder Work
page 68

Ladder Work

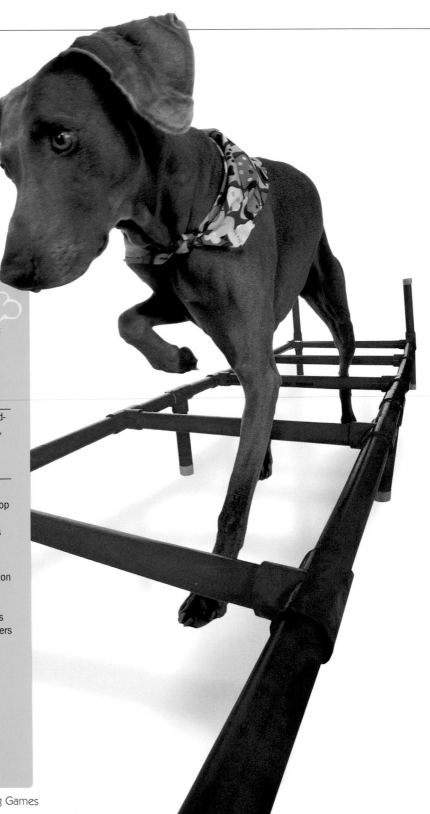

My front feet are easy. My back feet sometimes forget where to go.

Many dogs don't know they have back feet—their head leads them and everything else just follows. Ladder exercises teach your to work the mechanics of placing his feet.

TEACHING SKILLS:
Ladder work teaches coordination, hind-end awareness, balance, mental focus, and jumping skills.

PRIMARY USES:

SEARCH AND RESCUE
SAR dogs train on ladders to develop the hind-end awareness they will need to climb over fallen structures and debris.

AGILITY
Ladder training develops coordination for obstacles where the dog must space his steps and place all four feet quickly and accurately, such as the seesaw and the dogwalk. Ladders benefit dogs with contact-zone problems, teaching them to take small, controlled steps.

TRY IT:

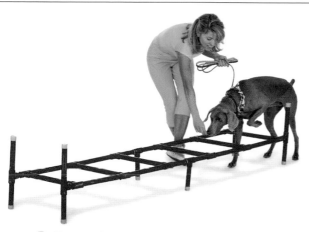

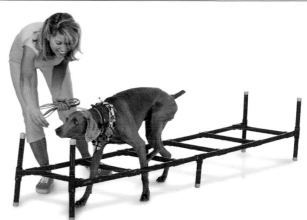

1 Place your ladder alongside a wall to prevent your dog from walking off the side. Use the hand closest to your dog to hold him on a short leash. In your other hand, hold several treats just above the ladder rung (keep your hand low so that your dog will be able to see where he is walking).

2 Lure your dog forward. After he has stepped through two or three rungs, give him one of the treats (always reward low, near the rungs). Continue luring him forward with another treat.

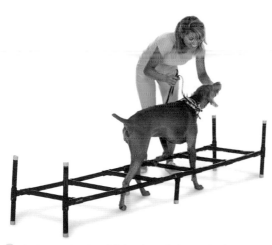

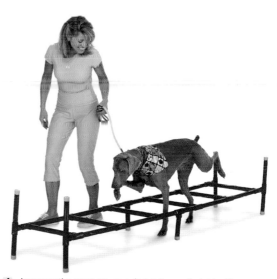

3 Turn around and switch hands so that your dog is now on the other side and go through again.

4 Increase the pace as your dog gets comfortable. Then move the ladder away from the wall and start over from the beginning.

TIP:	EQUIPMENT:	BUILD ON IT:
Some dogs may not even like to stand still with their feet between the rungs at first, so give your dog time. If your dog is sidestepping, squirming, or jumping, take him though the ladder more slowly.	A ladder is approximately 7 feet (2 m) long with rungs spaced 12 inches (30 cm) apart (used for any size dog). It stands a few inches off the ground but can be lowered by removing the legs for small dogs, puppies, or initial training.	Cavalettis *page 66* Bar Jump *page 104*

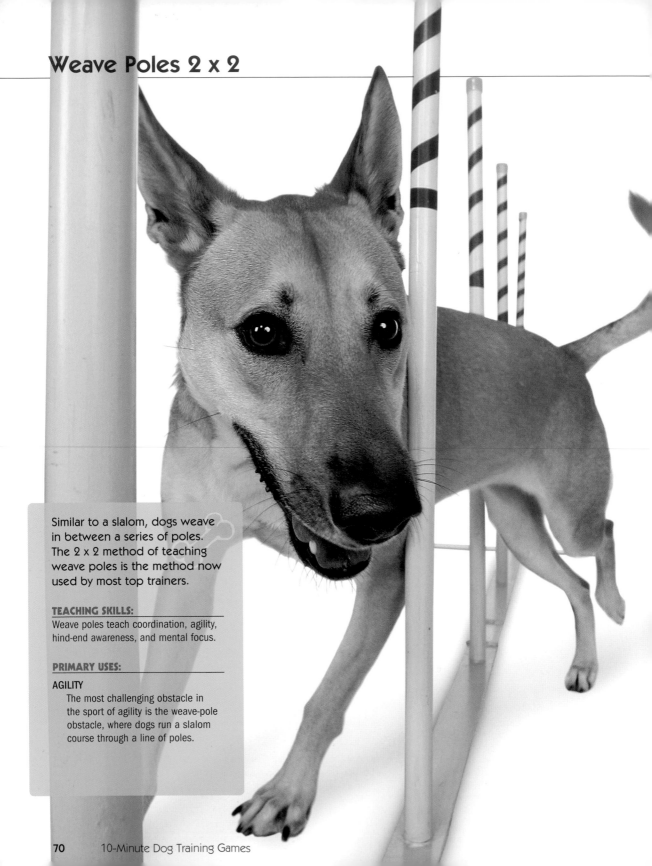

Weave Poles 2 x 2

Similar to a slalom, dogs weave in between a series of poles. The 2 x 2 method of teaching weave poles is the method now used by most top trainers.

TEACHING SKILLS:
Weave poles teach coordination, agility, hind-end awareness, and mental focus.

PRIMARY USES:

AGILITY
The most challenging obstacle in the sport of agility is the weave-pole obstacle, where dogs run a slalom course through a line of poles.

TRY IT:

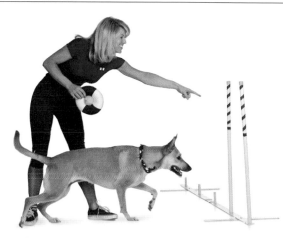

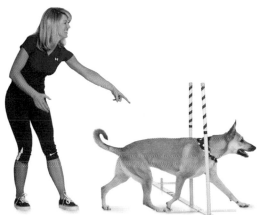

1 Start with just two poles. Send your dog through the poles any way you can, such as by using your pointed finger or a leash, or by running alongside the poles. Avoid luring your dog through with a treat.

2 The second your dog goes between the poles, toss a toy (or food toy) in FRONT of him. This will teach him to progress forward instead of turning back to look at you.

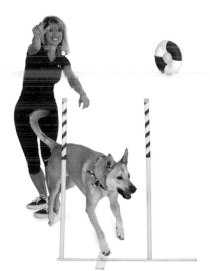

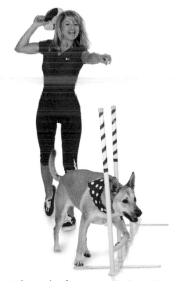

3 Once your dog has the hang of going between the poles, start to add more distance.

4 Now try to send your dog from an angle. In agility competition the dog must enter the set of poles with the first pole passing along his left shoulder.

TIP:	**EQUIPMENT:**	**BUILD ON IT:**
Once your dog has mastered two poles, add a second set of two poles in a parallel line, 15 feet (4.6 m) from the first set. Have your dog do one set and then the other set. Gradually move the two sets closer together.	Poles are about 3 feet (0.9 m) tall and spaced about 20 to 22 inches (51 to 56 cm) apart. PVC plastic pipe poles can be cut at an angle and pounded into the grass. Tall cones or plungers can be used as an indoor alternative.	Barrel Racing *page 142*

Paws-Up Balance Disc

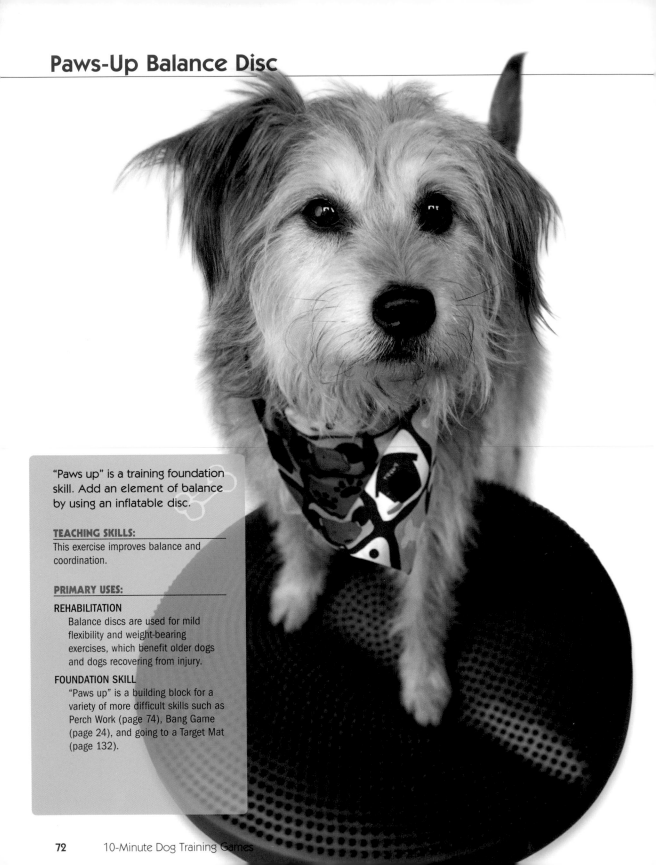

"Paws up" is a training foundation skill. Add an element of balance by using an inflatable disc.

TEACHING SKILLS:

This exercise improves balance and coordination.

PRIMARY USES:

REHABILITATION

Balance discs are used for mild flexibility and weight-bearing exercises, which benefit older dogs and dogs recovering from injury.

FOUNDATION SKILL

"Paws up" is a building block for a variety of more difficult skills such as Perch Work (page 74), Bang Game (page 24), and going to a Target Mat (page 132).

TRY IT:

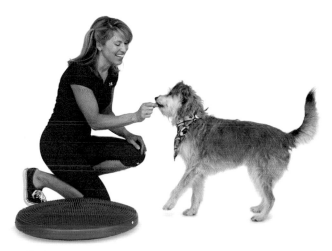

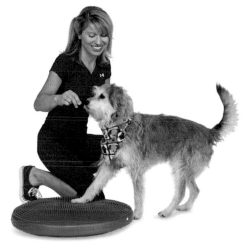

1 Get your dog's attention by holding a treat near his nose.

2 Slowly move the treat over the balance disc, luring your dog to put his front paws on it. Avoid moving your hand too fast, as your dog may jump over the disc.

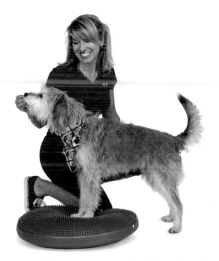

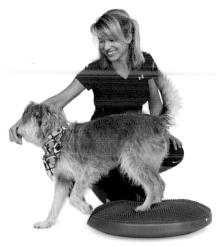

3 As soon as his paws come onto the disc, release the treat. It will be handy to hold several treats in your hand, so you can keep him in position by letting him sniff or lick another treat.

4 As an added challenge, lure your dog past the balance disc until his back paws come on, and his front paws come off.

TIP:

Most dogs can be lured onto a balance disc within a few minutes. As your dog improves, back your hand away for a few seconds, and then bring it forward to give him his treat. Give the treat only while your dog is in position—with his front paws on the balance disc.

EQUIPMENT:

Any low, stable object can be used for this exercise. An inflatable balance disc will give your dog an added challenge.

BUILD ON IT:

Perch Work
page 74

Skateboard
page 78

Perch Work

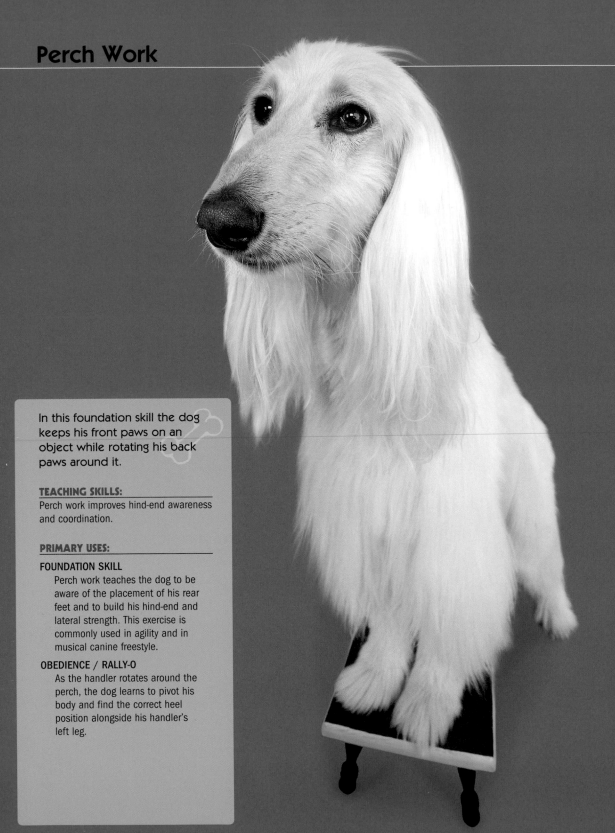

In this foundation skill the dog keeps his front paws on an object while rotating his back paws around it.

TEACHING SKILLS:
Perch work improves hind-end awareness and coordination.

PRIMARY USES:

FOUNDATION SKILL
Perch work teaches the dog to be aware of the placement of his rear feet and to build his hind-end and lateral strength. This exercise is commonly used in agility and in musical canine freestyle.

OBEDIENCE / RALLY-O
As the handler rotates around the perch, the dog learns to pivot his body and find the correct heel position alongside his handler's left leg.

TRY IT:

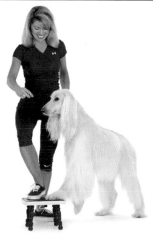

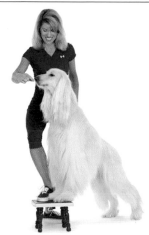

1 Hold a treat near your dog's nose and slowly bring it up above the perch. Your dog may try to walk around the perch or jump over it. Keep moving your treat slowly until he gets the idea to step on the perch with his front paws.

2 The instant his front paws come on the perch, release the treat. Allow him to nibble some additional treats in your hand while his paws remain on the perch.

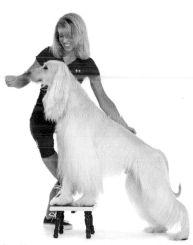

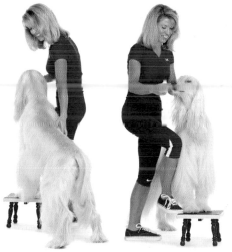

3 See if you can get your dog to rotate his back feet around the perch. Hold treats in front of his nose and use your other hand to gently nudge him sideways. The second he sidesteps with his rear feet, give him a treat.

4 Go slowly and try to get your dog to make one complete revolution.

TIP:

Perch work feels awkward for dogs at first, but they should quickly get the hang of it. It is important that you give the treat while your dog's paws are on the perch and not after he has come off. If he gets off the perch, just lure him back onto it.

EQUIPMENT:

A perch is about 1 foot (30 cm) in diameter, raised a few inches in height. Make a simple perch from a concrete brick, a cat litter pan, an upturned planter, a phone book, or other sturdy item.

BUILD ON IT:

Two On, Two Off
page 76

Peanut Roll
page 98

Two On, Two Off

Improve your dog's hind-end coordination by teaching him to place his back feet on a step.

TEACHING SKILLS:

This exercise builds your dog's hind-end awareness and coordination.

PRIMARY USES:

AGILITY

When dogs descend an inclined obstacle (or "contact obstacle") such as the seesaw, they are trained to pause at the bottom with their front feet on the ground and their back feet on the incline. Agility trainers call this the "two on, two off" method.

MUSICAL CANINE FREESTYLE

Dogs are taught to back up away from their handler by learning to place their back feet onto a step. The step is gradually moved farther and farther away from the handler.

TRY IT:

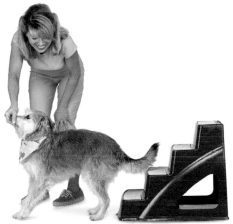

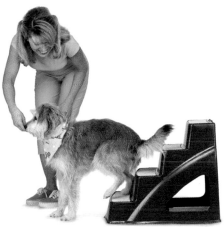

1 Set your steps next to a wall to confine your dog. Start with your dog directly in front of the steps. Hold a treat in your fist at your dog's nose height and slowly push the treat toward your dog's back feet. Use your body to crowd your dog so he doesn't veer to the side.

2 In an attempt to keep nibbling the treat, your dog may bow down a little, and will eventually back up. As soon as even one of his feet touches the step, mark that instant by saying, "Good!" and releasing the treat.

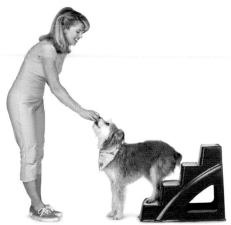

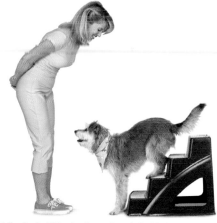

3 As your dog improves, try to get both of his hind feet to come onto the steps before you say, "Good!" and release the treat.

4 And finally, hold both of your hands behind your back and use your body to crowd your dog back onto the steps. The second his feet get on the steps, say, "Good!" and pull out the treat from behind your back.

TIP:	**EQUIPMENT:**	**BUILD ON IT:**
This exercise is an unusual behavior for your dog and requires a type of coordination not often used. You may see a lot of silly squirming at the beginning. Watch carefully so that you can give him the treat the instant one foot touches the step.	You can use a step, stairs of a staircase, an agility contact obstacle, a low perch, or a brick.	Ladder Climb *page 80* Seesaw *page 88*

Skateboard

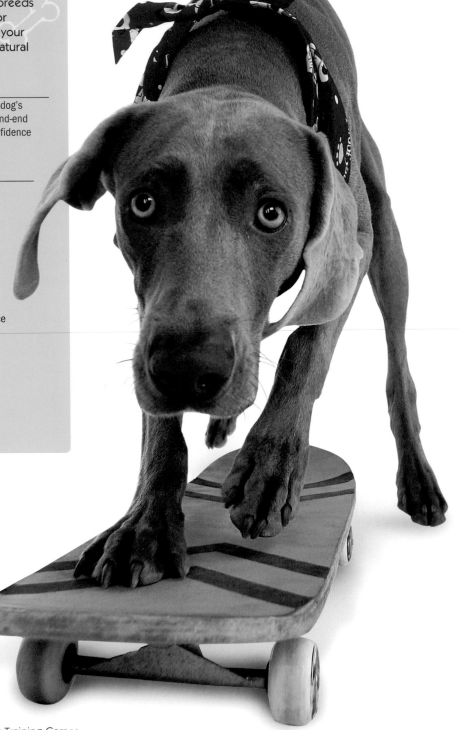

Some dogs (often bull breeds and terriers) go crazy for skateboards. Try it with your dog and see if he is a natural boarder!

TEACHING SKILLS:

Skateboarding improves your dog's balance, coordination, and hind-end awareness, as well as his confidence around strange noises.

PRIMARY USES:

EXERCISE

Some dogs really enjoy skateboarding and will play with their board for long periods of time on their own.

CUTE TRICK

If nothing else, a skateboarding dog is sure to bring a smile to the face of anyone who sees him!

TRY IT:

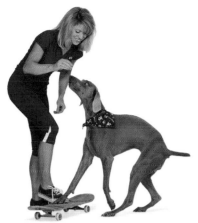

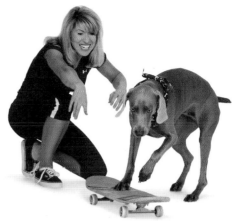

1 It's not uncommon for dogs to be initially scared of skateboard sounds, so start with the skateboard on carpet or grass, where it is quieter and moves slower. Put treats on the skateboard to encourage your dog to investigate it. Use a treat to lure him to put his front paws on it (see Paws-Up Balance Disc, page 72).

2 Roll the skateboard back and forth in front of your dog. If he moves toward it, roll it AWAY from your dog, so it runs away like a prey animal. Does he chase it? Praise your dog excitedly when he catches it, especially if he steps on it!

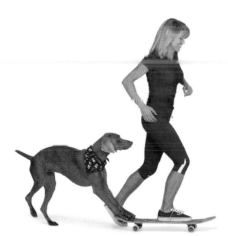

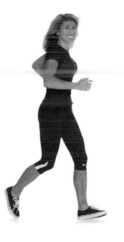

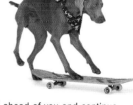

3 Take the skateboard to a parking lot and skate on it yourself. Call to your dog and encourage him to chase you. This can help engage his prey drive.

4 Run and toss the skateboard ahead of you and continue to chase it yourself. Use your voice to get your dog excited and chasing it too!

TIP:	EQUIPMENT:	BUILD ON IT:
Some dogs will have a natural drive to chase the skateboard and jump on top of it and often bite it as well. Few dogs love the skateboard on their first try, and most require at least several weeks of exposure to build drive for it.	Look for the largest-size skateboard that you can find. Very large dogs may need a specialty long board (a surf-board-inspired oversize board). You can make your own skateboard by attaching casters to the bottom of a foam body board or kickboard.	Wobble Board *page 94* Body Board *page 96*

Ladder Climb

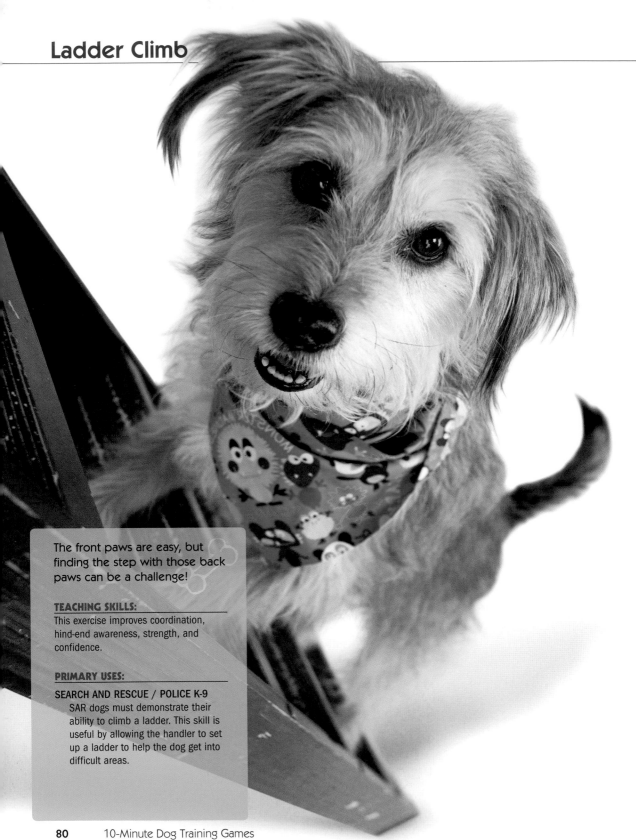

The front paws are easy, but finding the step with those back paws can be a challenge!

TEACHING SKILLS:

This exercise improves coordination, hind-end awareness, strength, and confidence.

PRIMARY USES:

SEARCH AND RESCUE / POLICE K-9

SAR dogs must demonstrate their ability to climb a ladder. This skill is useful by allowing the handler to set up a ladder to help the dog get into difficult areas.

TRY IT:

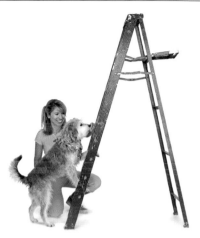

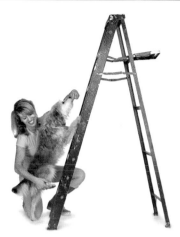

1 Hold a handful of treats and let your dog sniff them. Slowly raise your hand up the rungs of the ladder. Keep your eyes on your dog's front paws. The instant one paw touches a ladder rung, say, "Good!" and let him have a treat. Even if he doesn't touch the rung, you may need to occasionally give him a treat to keep his interest.

2 Continue to lure his head upward. The trickiest part is going to be getting your dog's first hind foot on the rung. As he struggles to find the rung, use your other hand to guide it in place.

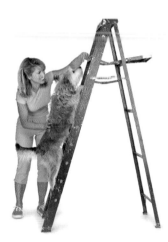

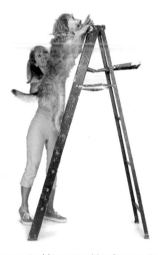

3 Keep luring your dog upward. Use your other hand to guard his body so that he doesn't fall.

4 Have an extra-big treat waiting for your dog at the top of the ladder.

TIP:

Practice no more than five minutes per session, as this exercise is mentally and physically tiring for your dog. Always lift your dog off the ladder rather than allowing him to jump off, as he could injure himself in jumping.

EQUIPMENT:

For SAR work, the ladder must be 6 to 8 feet (1.8 to 2.4 m) high with flat rungs. The ladder is secured at a 45-degree angle. Apply grip tape to the steps to provide traction.

BUILD ON IT:

Ladder Work
page 68

Ramp

Climbing a ramp can be scary at first, but with a little help, your dog will be zooming up and down in no time!

TEACHING SKILLS:
Walking a ramp will increase your dog's balance, coordination, and confidence.

PRIMARY USES:

AGILITY
A ramp is located at either end of the agility dogwalk obstacle. The A-frame obstacle is two steep ramps.

SENIOR DOGS
As a dog ages, he may require a ramp to get into and out of a car, or onto furniture. Teach him this skill before the need arises.

SEARCH AND RESCUE
SAR dogs must be able to climb a 12-inch (30 cm) wide ramp up a height of 3 feet (0.9 m).

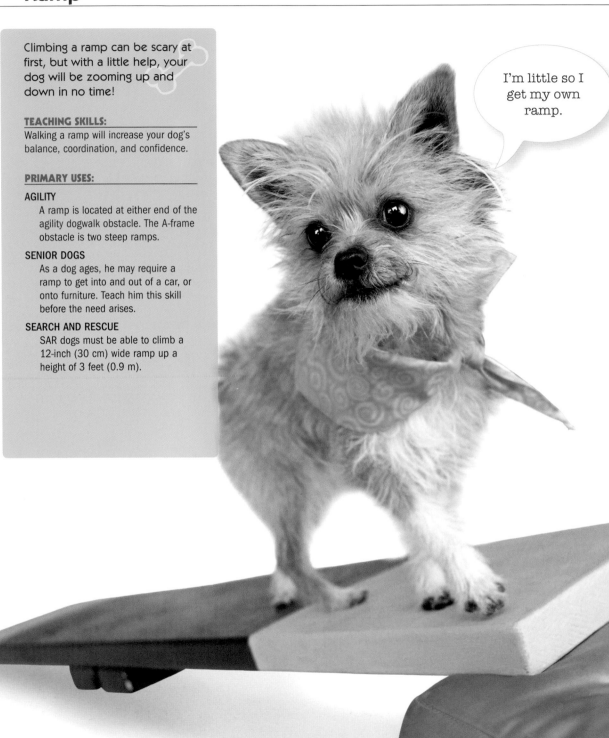

I'm little so I get my own ramp.

TRY IT:

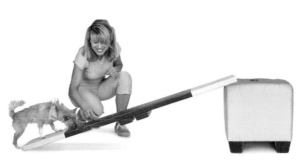

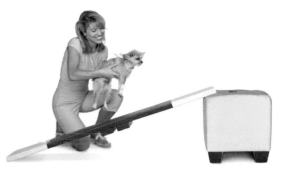

1 Rest a ramp securely on an armchair or sofa, up against a wall. Place a line of closely spaced treats up the ramp (dabs of peanut butter or sliced deli meat won't roll off). Position your body on the side of the ramp to discourage your dog from jumping off the side. Point out the first treat to him.

2 When your dog is halfway up the ramp, he may decide he wants to get off. Do not allow him to jump off the side, as this can be dangerous, and you don't want your dog to develop this bad habit. Instead, if he looks anxious, simply lift him off the ramp and onto the floor.

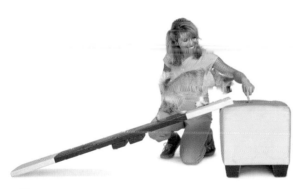

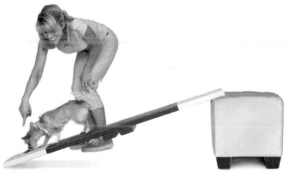

3 Keep adding treats along the ramp until your dog makes it all the way to the top. When he does, give him a big dog biscuit!

4 Once your dog has the hang of going up the ramp, repeat the process to teach him to walk down the ramp. Your dog will be tempted to jump off the side, so place a big treat at the base of the ramp and point it out to him.

TIP:	EQUIPMENT:	BUILD ON IT:
As with any feared object, it is important that you don't push your dog past his comfort level, as this would only increase his fear. The fastest way to have him overcome his fear is to allow him to approach the item on his own terms and be able to escape when he wants to.	Pet ramps that secure to a car entrance are widely available and have a nonslip surface. Make your own ramp by fastening carpet or grip tape to a board.	Balance Beam *page 84* Seesaw *page 88*

Balance Beam

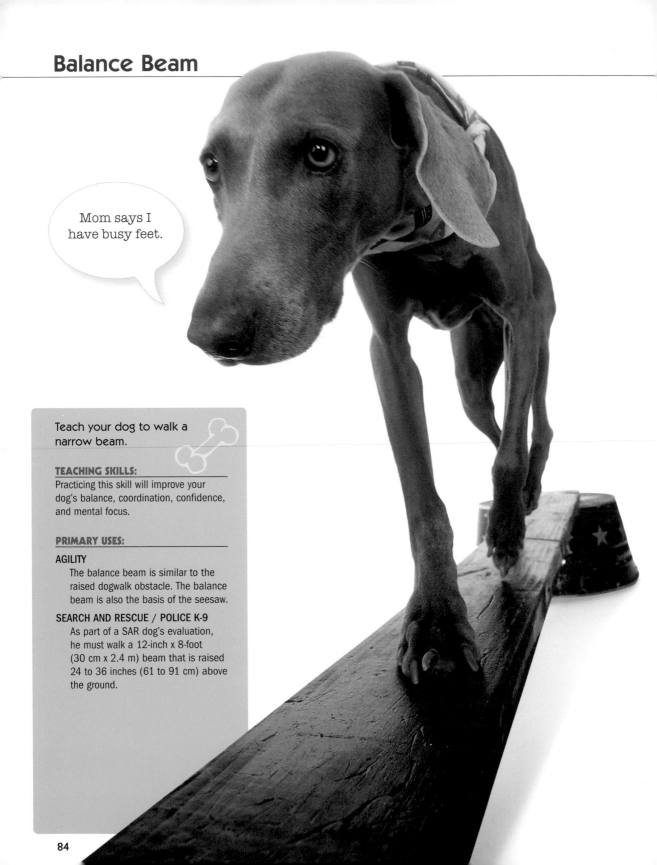

Mom says I have busy feet.

Teach your dog to walk a narrow beam.

TEACHING SKILLS:

Practicing this skill will improve your dog's balance, coordination, confidence, and mental focus.

PRIMARY USES:

AGILITY

The balance beam is similar to the raised dogwalk obstacle. The balance beam is also the basis of the seesaw.

SEARCH AND RESCUE / POLICE K-9

As part of a SAR dog's evaluation, he must walk a 12-inch x 8-foot (30 cm x 2.4 m) beam that is raised 24 to 36 inches (61 to 91 cm) above the ground.

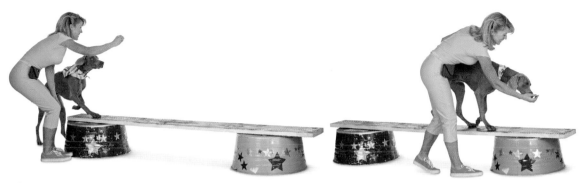

1 Construct a sturdy balance beam of a height somewhere between your dog's elbows and withers (shoulders). Place the beam against a wall to block your dog from jumping off. Hold a handful of treats and use one to lure your dog up onto the end of the beam. Give him a treat once he is on the beam.

2 Continue to move a treat forward, drawing your dog along with it. Keep your hand low so your dog can still see the beam. Use your body to block your dog from jumping off (don't touch your dog, but position your body adjacent to him). Give him a treat every few steps.

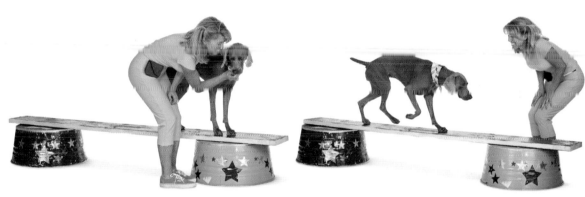

3 Make it a habit to always have your dog walk the entire beam, exiting at the far end rather than jumping off at the middle. This allows you to control his exit and reduce the risk of injury.

4 Over time, phase out the treats you were giving him in the middle of the beam but continue to give him a treat at the end.

TIP:	EQUIPMENT:	BUILD ON IT:
Over time, you can go to a skinnier beam. Decrease the beam width in small increments of about 2 inches (5 cm) or your dog will become confused.	Construct a balance beam from a plank affixed to two concrete blocks or crates. Adhere carpet, grip tape, or skid-guard paint to the beam for extra traction. Improvise a balance beam by laying six concrete blocks in a line, or by utilizing a low garden wall or picnic bench.	Double Beam /Tightrope *page 86*

Double Beam / Tightrope

Challenge your dog's coordination by having him walk across a split beam.

TEACHING SKILLS:
This challenging exercise requires balance, coordination, confidence, and mental focus.

PRIMARY USES:

TRICKS
Walking a tightrope is a traditional circus dog trick. Over time, the two beams are replaced with two taut cables.

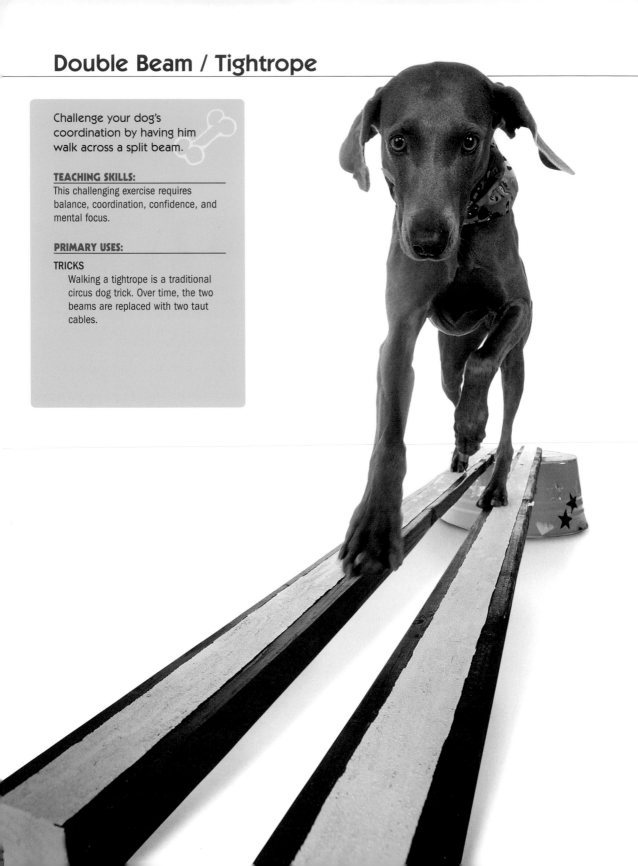

TRY IT:

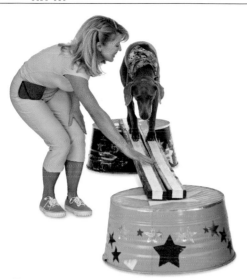

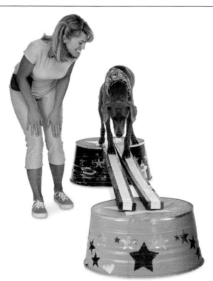

1 First, teach your dog to walk a Balance Beam (page 84). Next, replace your balance beam with two 2 x 4-inch (5 x 10 cm) boards. Press the two boards together securely, so they appear as a single board. Have your dog walk to the beam and reward him at the end.

2 Arrange the boards in a *V* with the boards pressed together at the "start" end, and separated by 2 inches (5 cm) at the "finish" end. This *V* makes enough of a change in the boards to cause your dog to look down and figure out where to place his feet.

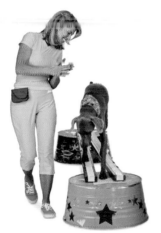

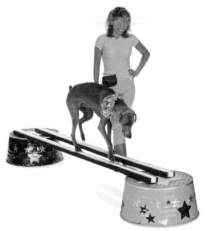

3 Widen the *V* so that the boards are separated even farther on the "finish" end.

4 Finally, make both beams parallel and separated so that they are shoulder width apart for your dog.

TIP:	EQUIPMENT:	BUILD ON IT:

TIP:

If your dog ever falls, don't end the session with him being scared. Ask him for something easy, such as putting just his front paws on the beam, and end the session with that small success.

EQUIPMENT:

Use two parallel 8-foot (2.4 m) long 2 x 4-inch (5 x 10 cm) boards and secure them to wooden crates. Attach grip tape or paint them with traction paint. The boards should be elevated no higher than your dog's armpit, as your dog could potentially slip and straddle the board.

BUILD ON IT:

Ladder Climb
page 80

Balance Ball
page 102

Seesaw

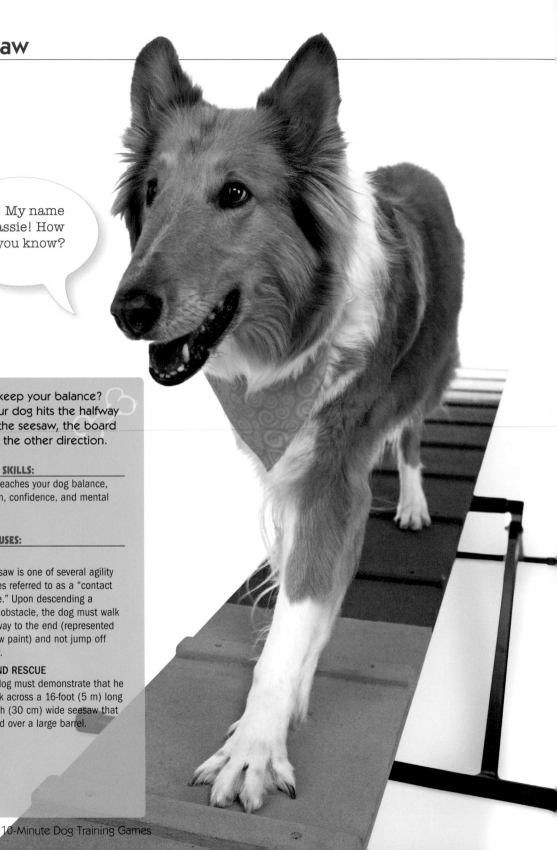

Yes! My name *is* Lassie! How did you know?

Can you keep your balance? When your dog hits the halfway point of the seesaw, the board will tip in the other direction.

TEACHING SKILLS:

This game teaches your dog balance, coordination, confidence, and mental focus.

PRIMARY USES:

AGILITY

The seesaw is one of several agility obstacles referred to as a "contact obstacle." Upon descending a contact obstacle, the dog must walk all the way to the end (represented by yellow paint) and not jump off mid-way.

SEARCH AND RESCUE

A SAR dog must demonstrate that he can walk across a 16-foot (5 m) long x 12-inch (30 cm) wide seesaw that is placed over a large barrel.

TRY IT:

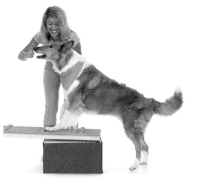

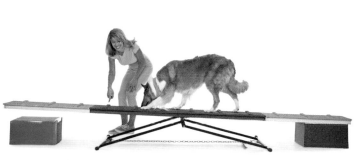

1 It will be helpful to first practice Wobble Board (page 94), Bang Game (page 24), Ramp (page 82), and Balance Beam (page 84). If your seesaw has an adjustable fulcrum, set it to the lowest level. Otherwise, position a platform under one or both ends of the board. Use a treat to lure your dog onto the board.

2 Lay treats along the board, just ahead of your dog. Space the treats very closely together near the middle of the seesaw, because you want your dog to move slowly when the seesaw pivots. If your dog jumps off the board, bring him to the start and have him get back on from the end rather than from the middle.

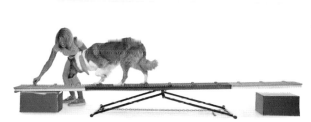

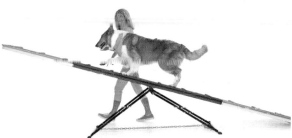

3 Always place a treat at the very end of the seesaw to create a habit in your dog of slowing down at the end instead of leaping off (which could be dangerous).

4 Very gradually raise the fulcrum or lower the platforms. Walk along the seesaw next to your dog to keep him focused and to prevent him from jumping off the side.

TIP:

It is not uncommon for dogs to be fearful of the seesaw at first. Even after they have walked the seesaw they may have periods of regressing back to fearfulness. Never push your dog to do more than he is comfortable with, as that would increase his fear. Take it slow and use lots of tasty treats.

EQUIPMENT:

A regulation agility seesaw is 12 feet (3.7 m) long, 12 inches (30 cm) wide, and has a fulcrum 24 inches (61 cm) high. The board has traction bumps and a nonskid painted surface.

BUILD ON IT:

Two On, Two Off
page 76

Balance Beam
page 84

Stacking Pods

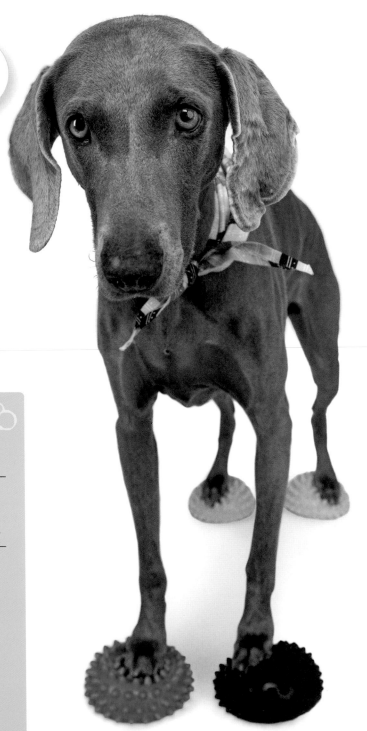

Practice "stacking" by having your dog balance with each foot on a pod.

TEACHING SKILLS:

This exercise challenges your dog's balance, coordination, hind-end awareness, and mental focus.

PRIMARY USES:

CONFORMATION DOG SHOW

In conformation competition dogs must "stack," or stand squarely, so that a judge can evaluate their structure. Pods are used in training to set the dog's feet in the proper position.

TRY IT:

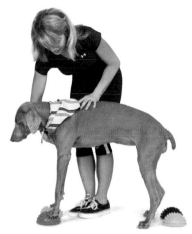

1 Lift your dog's chest until his front feet are off the ground, and then lower him slowly down. His feet will naturally come down at the proper width apart, so have your pods set with similar spacing.

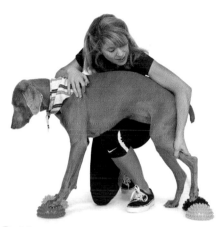

2 Adjust one back foot at a time by lifting each from above the hock.

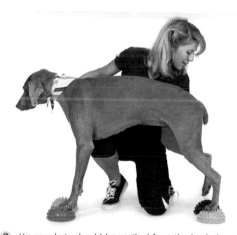

3 His rear legs should be vertical from the hock down.

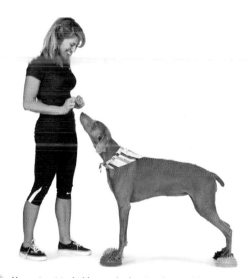

4 Use a treat to hold your dog's attention and keep him still.

TIP:

This exercise can be tougher than it looks! With squirmy dogs, work with only the front paws to start. Over time your dog can learn to place his feet himself!

EQUIPMENT:

Four bricks or heavy books make perfect pods for a dog to stand on.

BUILD ON IT:

Donut
page 92

Donut

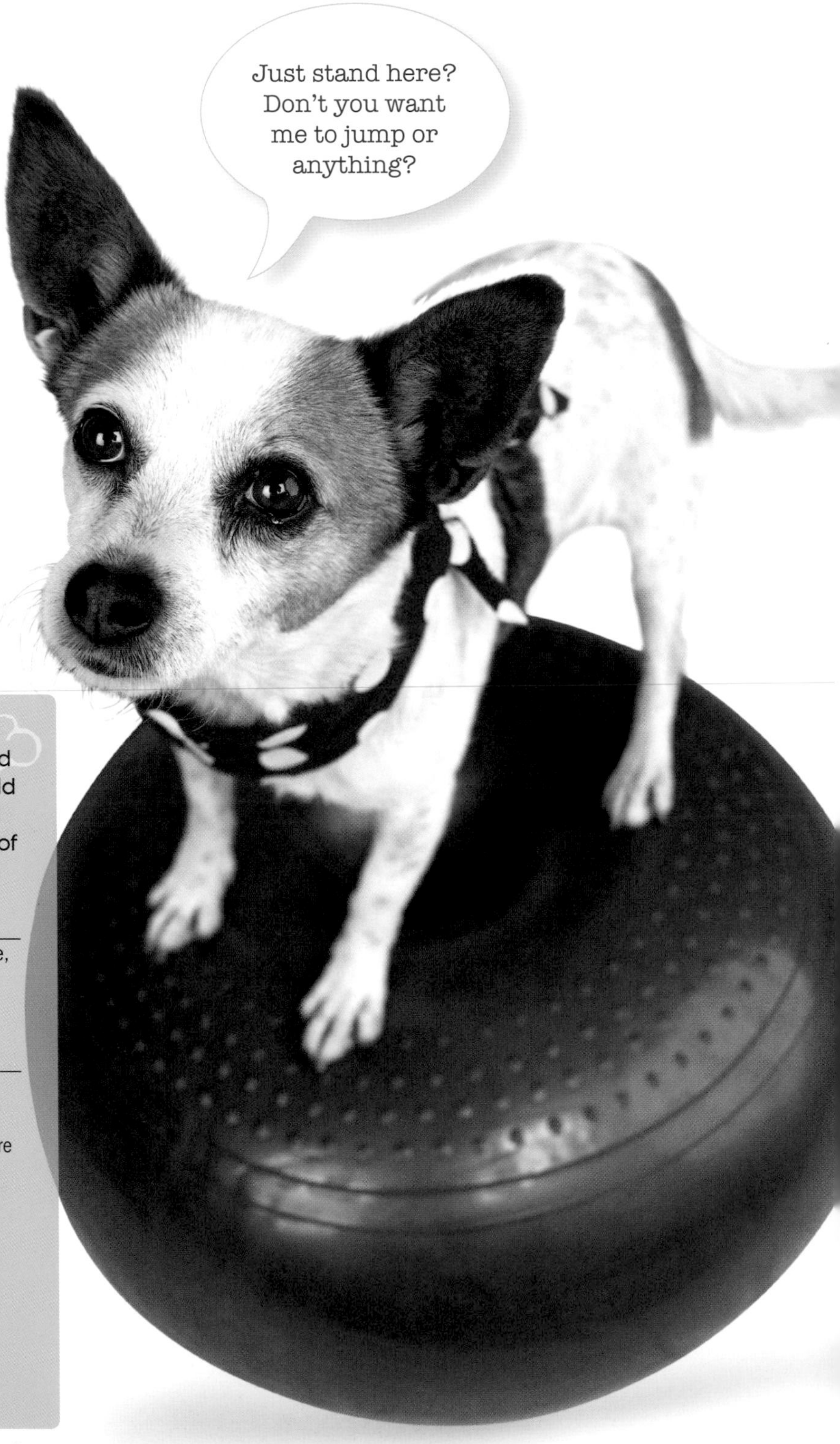

Just stand here? Don't you want me to jump or anything?

When his weight shifts, your dog's balance is challenged and his muscles are tensed. This mild exercise improves balance and can be used for rehabilitation of injured joints and muscles.

TEACHING SKILLS:

The donut improves your dog's balance, coordination, confidence, and mental focus.

PRIMARY USES:

FITNESS & REHABILITATION

A variety of shapes and sizes of inflatable cushions are used for core strengthening and weight-bearing therapy for older or injured dogs. As he shifts his weight, the dog's muscles are put gently through a range of motions and stresses.

TRY IT:

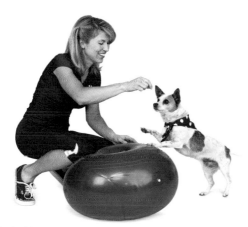

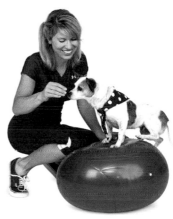

1 Stabilize the donut with your knee. Hold several treats in your hand and slowly move your hand from your dog's nose up over the donut. In reaching for the treat your dog should put his front paws on the donut. Let him have a the treat and keep him there by letting him sniff the other treats in your hand.

2 As your dog nibbles treats from your hand, slowly move your hand farther across the donut, prompting your dog to climb after it.

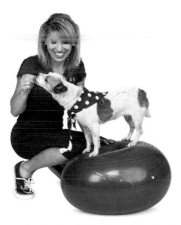

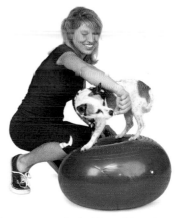

3 When your dog is standing on top of the donut, allow him to nibble more treats. Keep your other hand close to him and be ready to stabilize him if he starts to fall.

4 Move your treat slowly side to side, or in a complete circle, guiding him along. He will need to balance as he shifts his weight and moves after the treat.

TIP:	EQUIPMENT:	BUILD ON IT:
Although they may be hesitant at first, most dogs grow to love this game. When not in use, you may have to hide the donut away, lest your dog jump on top of it on his own!	Specially-made dog balance cushions are made from heavy-duty PVC material that resists damage caused by dogs' nails. Cushions often have traction bumps on the top side.	Balance Ball *page 102*

Wobble Board

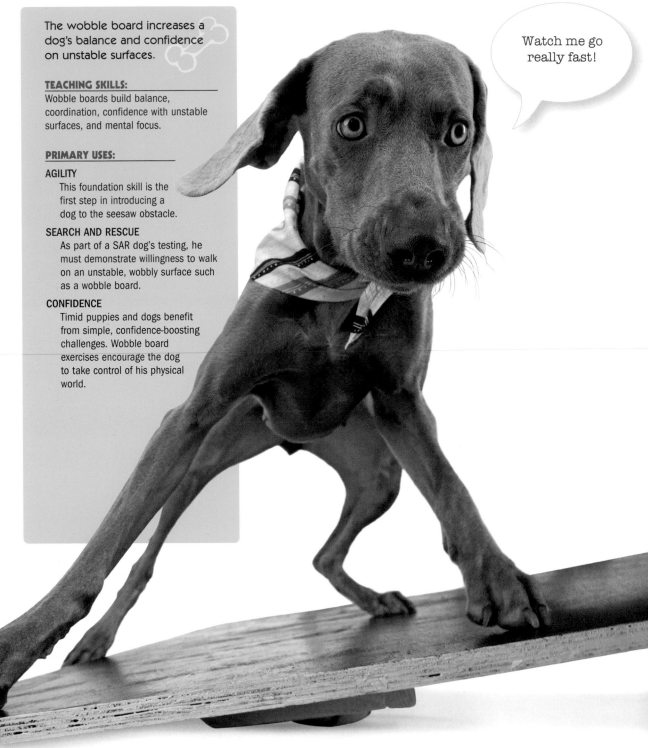

The wobble board increases a dog's balance and confidence on unstable surfaces.

TEACHING SKILLS:
Wobble boards build balance, coordination, confidence with unstable surfaces, and mental focus.

PRIMARY USES:

AGILITY
This foundation skill is the first step in introducing a dog to the seesaw obstacle.

SEARCH AND RESCUE
As part of a SAR dog's testing, he must demonstrate willingness to walk on an unstable, wobbly surface such as a wobble board.

CONFIDENCE
Timid puppies and dogs benefit from simple, confidence-boosting challenges. Wobble board exercises encourage the dog to take control of his physical world.

Watch me go really fast!

TRY IT:

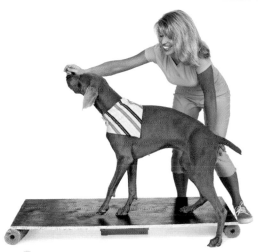

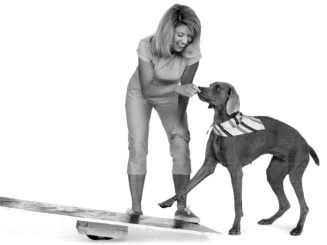

1 Place the wobble board on grass or carpeting to lessen the bang noise, and immobilize it with blocks or foam noodles under the edges. Place your dog's food dish on the board to get him used to it. Use a treat to lure your dog to step on the board and give him the treat while he has at least one paw on the board.

2 Remove the supports from under the board. Step on one end of the board to make it less wobbly. This gradual change allows your dog to know it is unsteady and know that he controls whether it moves. Continue to use a treat to lure your dog to step on it.

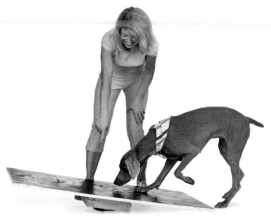

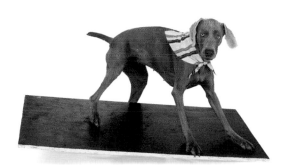

3 Place some treats on the board and point them out to your dog, encouraging him to walk on the board to get them.

4 Later, just point to the board and see if your dog will step on it. When he does, give him a treat from your pocket.

EQUIPMENT:

The board is made from ³/₄-inch (2 cm) plywood. A **rocker board** rocks in only one direction (like a seesaw). The 44 x 22-inch (1 m x 56 cm) board has a plastic pipe secured along its center. A **wobble board** is a 3 to 4-foot (1 to 1.2 m) square or a circle with universal rotation. A long screw is driven through the board and into a softball. A **buja board** (pictured) has a small square of 2 x 4-inch (5 x 10 cm) boards attached to its underside. Place a ball inside the square.

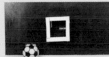

BUILD ON IT:

Seesaw
page 88

Body Board
page 96

Body Board

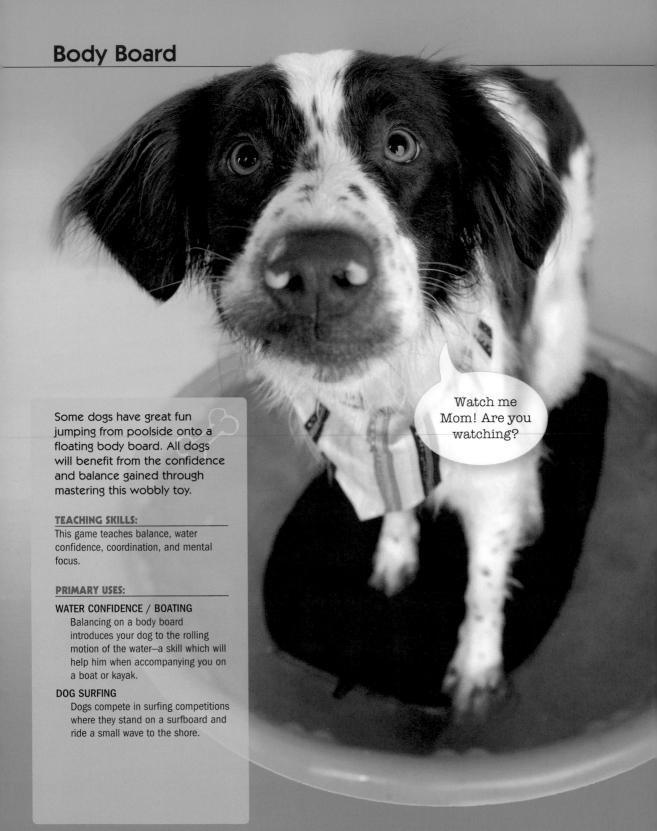

Some dogs have great fun jumping from poolside onto a floating body board. All dogs will benefit from the confidence and balance gained through mastering this wobbly toy.

TEACHING SKILLS:

This game teaches balance, water confidence, coordination, and mental focus.

PRIMARY USES:

WATER CONFIDENCE / BOATING

Balancing on a body board introduces your dog to the rolling motion of the water—a skill which will help him when accompanying you on a boat or kayak.

DOG SURFING

Dogs compete in surfing competitions where they stand on a surfboard and ride a small wave to the shore.

TRY IT:

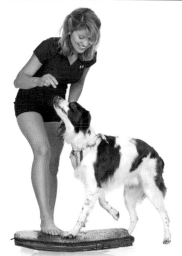

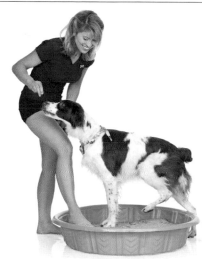

1 Dogs are going to be naturally wary of this unfamiliar toy. Introduce your dog to the body board on dry land. Use a treat to lure him to step on it and let him nibble the treat while he has one or more paws on the board.

2 Put the body board in an empty wading pool. Again, use a treat to lure your dog to step on it and let him nibble the treat there.

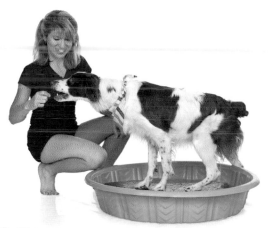

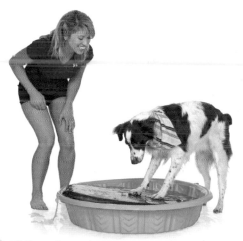

3 Fill the wading pool with just a few inches of water and lure your dog just as you did before. If your dog is wary, try the Weenie Bobbing game (page 14) to increase his water confidence.

4 Fill the wading pool with more water. Encourage your dog to jump and splash on the board to increase his confidence.

TIP:

Some dogs will be reluctant to get even their paws wet. Use extra-tempting treats such as chicken, steak, or cheese. Never force or place your dog into the water, as that could easily make him even more fearful. It's better to take it slowly, even if it takes several sessions before your dog places his first paw in the water.

EQUIPMENT:

Body boards (also called boogie boards, kickboards, or foam boards) come in a variety of sizes and buoyancies. Larger boards will be easiest for your dog.

BUILD ON IT:

Donut
page 92

Wobble
Board
page 94

Peanut Roll

Your dog uses his front paws to roll an inflatable peanut-shaped cylinder.

TEACHING SKILLS:

This game will improve your dog's balance, coordination, and strength.

PRIMARY USES:

FITNESS & REHABILITATION

Different shapes of inflatable stability balls are used for core conditioning and weight-bearing therapy for injured dogs. Having the dog shift his weight puts his muscles through a range of motions and gentle stresses.

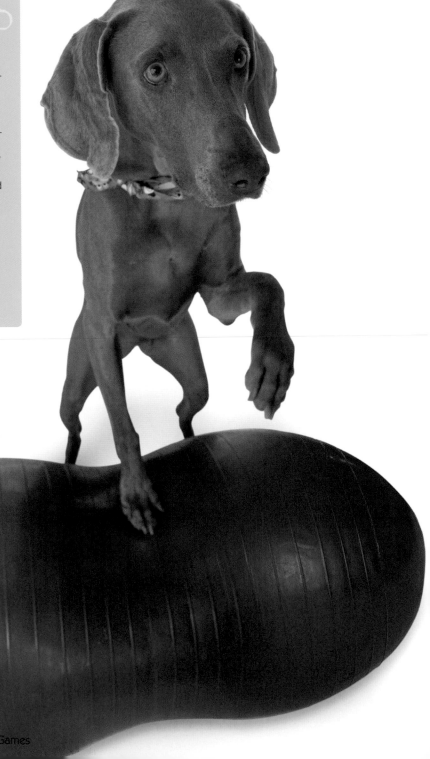

TRY IT:

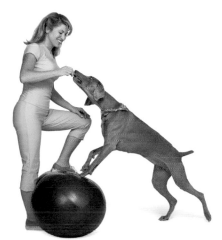

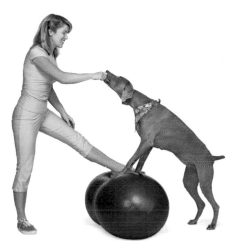

1 Hold the peanut ball steady with your knee and foot. Hold a handful of treats and slowly move them from your dog's nose, up, over the peanut. Your dog should put his front paws on the peanut as he reaches for the treat.

2 Keep your dog's attention by letting him continue to sniff and nibble the treats in your hand. Keeping your foot on the peanut and back up your other foot in preparation for rolling the peanut.

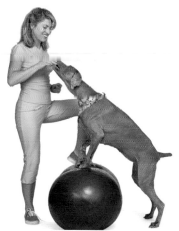

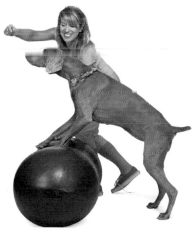

3 Use your foot to roll the peanut slowly toward you. The second that your dog adjusts either of his front feet, say, "Good!" and release your treat. Back up and roll the peanut again.

4 As your dog improves, he will be able to roll the peanut more and more by himself, and you can move to his side (still helping to roll the peanut with your hand).

TIP:	EQUIPMENT:	BUILD ON IT:
Dogs quickly learn to put their front paws on the peanut, but the coordination and logic required to roll it is more difficult. Focus on helping your dog maintain control and steady posture, which will benefit his strength training.	Dog stability balls come in a variety of sizes. The peanut-shaped ball limits movement to front/back, making it easier for your dog to learn to roll it.	Barrel *page 100* Balance Ball *page 102*

Barrel

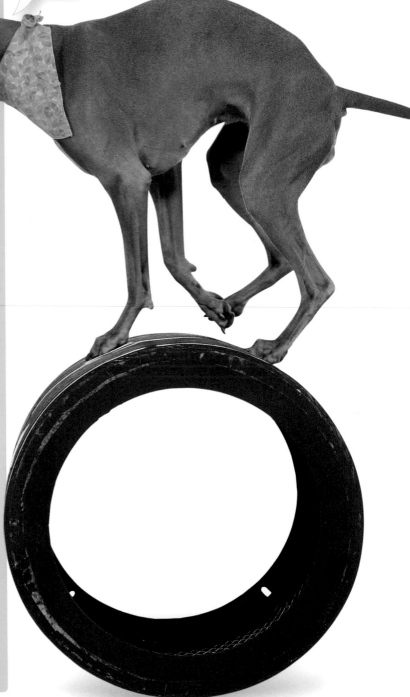

Because that's the way I roll . . .

Rolling a barrel will be challenging for your dog as he learns to control his balance and place his feet deliberately.

TEACHING SKILLS:

This exercise will challenge your dog's balance, coordination, strength, and mental focus.

PRIMARY USES:

TRICK

Rolling on a barrel is a traditional circus dog trick.

SCHUTZHUND

In Schutzhund training and competition, dogs must climb over barrels that are placed as obstacles in their path.

SEARCH AND RESCUE / POLICE K-9

As a training exercise, three barrels are stacked in a pyramid for dogs to scale.

GUN DOGS

Barrel work is used in training hunting dogs to "whoa" (stop and remain still). The dog stands on the barrel while the trainer steadies it. If the dog moves around or diverts his attention, the trainer allows the barrel to wobble. In this way, the dog learns to stay focused and still.

TRY IT:

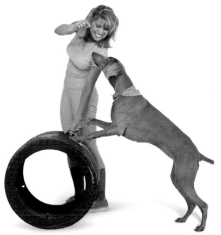

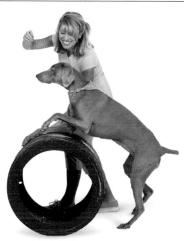

1 Place the barrel against a wall or use your hand to hold it still. Hold a treat above the barrel to lure your dog to put his front paws up. Give him a treat when his paws come up and encourage him to stay there by continuing to give him small treats every few seconds.

2 Once your dog is confident, hold a treat in front of your dog to keep his attention and use your other hand to roll the barrel away from your dog a few inches. Every time he repositions a paw, say, "Good!" and give him a treat.

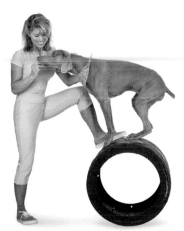

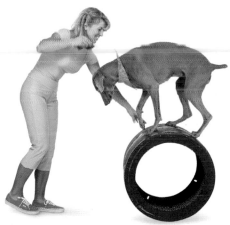

3 Stand on the opposite side of the barrel and hold it with your knee or foot. Use a handful of treats to lure your dog on top of the barrel. As he tries to steady himself he may press against your hand, which is fine.

4 Very slowly, roll the barrel a few inches backward, so that your dog has to take a step forward. Keep your hand with the treats by his nose and give him a treat every few seconds.

TIP:	EQUIPMENT:	BUILD ON IT:

This is a challenging skill for any dog, so give your dog lots of praise and treats to keep him motivated. Avoid physically holding your dog on the barrel, as he will likely feel more secure if he knows he can jump off. Your dog may need weeks or months to feel steady on the barrel.

Construct a barrel from a 55-gallon (208 L) plastic drum (sold at horse feed stores.) Cover the barrel with rubber matting or carpet, secured in place with glue. Use duct tape around the edges. Little dogs can use smaller plastic drums.

Peanut Roll
page 98

Balance Ball
page 102

Balance Ball

Balance-ball work develops core strength and muscle tone as well as balance, range of motion, and flexibility.

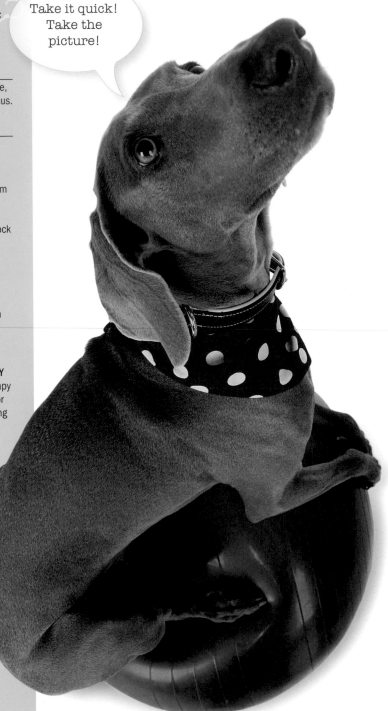

Take it quick! Take the picture!

TEACHING SKILLS:

This game improves your dog's balance, strength, coordination, and mental focus.

PRIMARY USES:

PERFORMANCE SPORTS

Performance dogs are at risk for lower- and mid-back problems and muscle strains, and will benefit from core-strengthening exercises. Ball work is commonly used for canine athletes in agility, lure coursing, dock jumping, and herding.

SENIOR DOGS

The first place we see weakness as dogs age is in their hind end and lower back. Ball work is an effective and safe way to condition these muscles, which will aid in the reduction and prevention of problems.

REHABILITATION / PHYSICAL THERAPY

Ball work is used as physical therapy for dogs recuperating from injury or surgery. It provides gentle stretching and strengthening opportunities.

TRY IT:

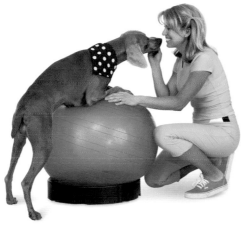

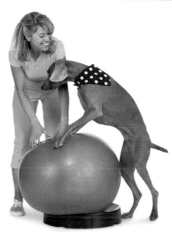

1 Hold the balance ball steady or set it on a ball stabilizer. Move a treat from your dog's nose, over the ball, to get him to place his forelegs on the ball. Let him sniff and nibble treats in your hand to keep him in position. Gently rock the ball back and forth so that he uses his rear legs to balance.

2 Walk around the ball to encourage your dog to sidestep and pivot around the ball (see Perch Work, page 74).

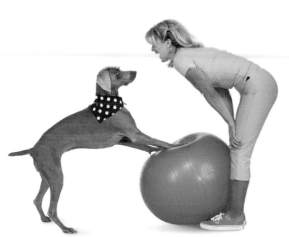

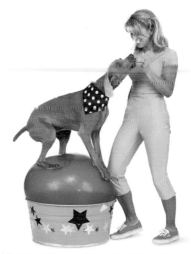

3 Remove the ball stabilizer and allow the ball to wobble under your dog. Encourage him to experiment with it and praise him and give him treats for confident behavior.

4 Stabilize the ball in a box or strap it to a tire. Lure your dog to climb on top of the ball. After a few seconds give him a treat and have him come off the ball.

TIP:

Once dogs realize that they gets treats for interacting with the balance ball, they often bounce on it happily! Keep your older or injured dog in control and moving slowly when interacting with the ball.

EQUIPMENT:

Canine balance balls (also called physioballs or theraballs) are tougher than the ones made for humans, which can be punctured by dogs' nails. Canine balance balls come in a variety of sizes. The larger the ball, and the more inflated it is, the easier it will be to balance on.

BUILD ON IT:

Stacking Pods
page 90

Peanut Roll
page 98

Bar Jump

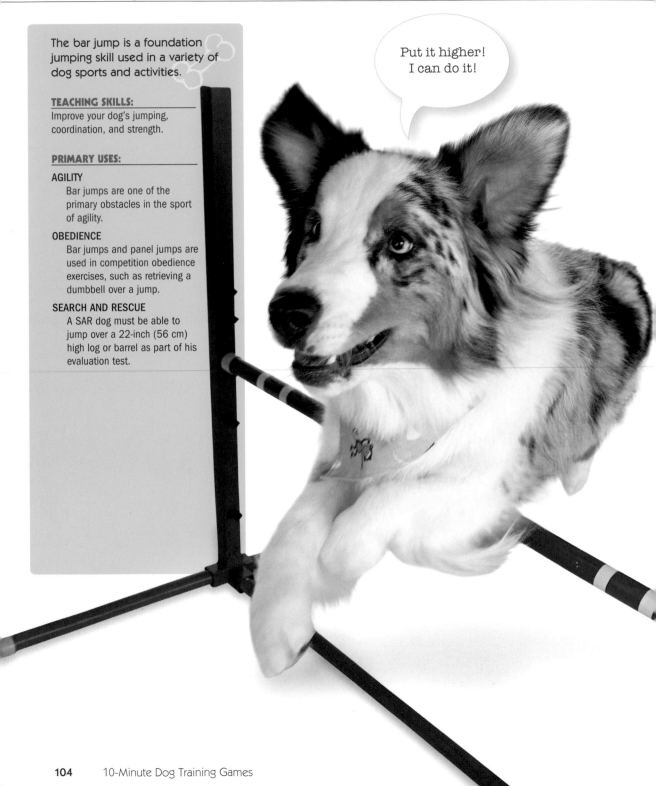

The bar jump is a foundation jumping skill used in a variety of dog sports and activities.

TEACHING SKILLS:
Improve your dog's jumping, coordination, and strength.

PRIMARY USES:

AGILITY
Bar jumps are one of the primary obstacles in the sport of agility.

OBEDIENCE
Bar jumps and panel jumps are used in competition obedience exercises, such as retrieving a dumbbell over a jump.

SEARCH AND RESCUE
A SAR dog must be able to jump over a 22-inch (56 cm) high log or barrel as part of his evaluation test.

Put it higher! I can do it!

TRY IT:

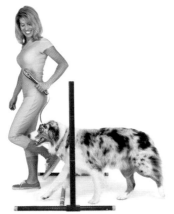

1 Set the bar on the ground between the two stanchions. With your dog on a lead, walk with him between the stanchions a few times, and then jog between the stanchions. Praise him and give him a treat to keep him motivated.

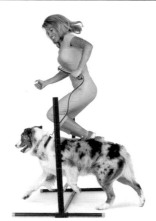

2 Set the bar to a low height, approximately half the height of your dog's elbows. Jog with him toward the jump and give an enthusiastic "hup!" as you jump over the bar with him. Continue to praise and treat him every time.

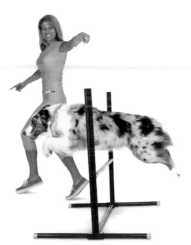

3 Gradually raise the bar and try running alongside the jump instead of over it. Extend your arm to guide your dog toward the center of the jump (pretend you are holding an invisible leash).

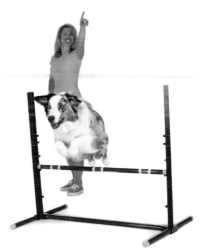

4 Experiment with starting your dog farther from the jump, or at an angle to teach him to find the jump from wherever he is.

TIP:	EQUIPMENT:	BUILD ON IT:
During the transition between your running over the jump and running alongside it, your dog may try to sneak around the side of the jump. You can position the jump alongside a wall to prevent this.	Construct a bar jump from PVC plastic pipes and connectors. Jump cups (sold at dog agility venues) snap onto the poles and allow the bar to roll off if your dog knocks it. Jump heights vary per sport and organization. A standard jump height equals the dog's height at his withers (shoulders) plus or minus 2 inches (5 cm).	Stride Regulators *page 106*

Stride Regulators

Set-point exercises teach a dog to judge distance, and to place his stride and collect his body at the proper distance in front of a jump for maximum jumping efficiency

TEACHING SKILLS:
This foundation exercise improves jumping skill, coordination, and strength.

PRIMARY USES:

AGILITY
Stride regulators teach a dog to read distance and control his body accordingly. The dog learns appropriate takeoff place, weight transfer, angle of elevation, and height evaluation. Stride-regulator exercises teach dogs how to best collect themselves before a jump for maximum height.

FLYBALL
Stride-regulator exercises teach a dog to think about his stride when approaching hurdles.

DOCK DIVING
A diving dog that stutter-steps or takes off too far in front of the dock edge is losing distance. Stride-regulator exercises teach the dog to judge distance and alter his stride accordingly.

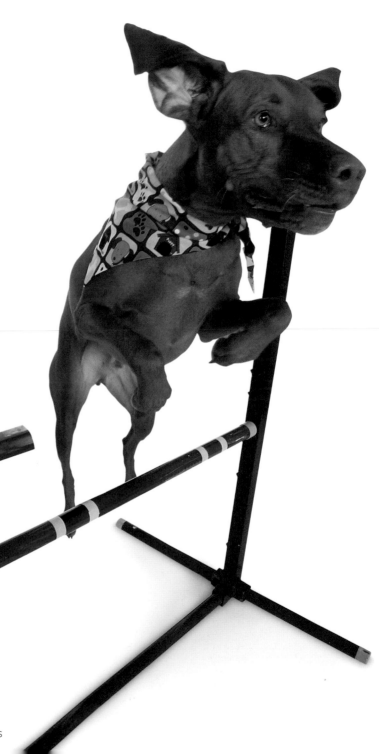

TRY IT:

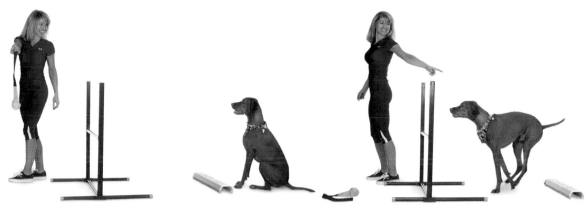

1 First, teach your dog the Bar Jump (page 104). The jump bump defines the takeoff spot and work area. Set your dog directly behind the jump bump. Walk past the bar jump and drop your dog's favorite toy on the ground. The toy is used to train your dog to drive toward a target.

2 Release your dog to jump. Your dog should bounce (hit the ground only once). At the point where the bounce occurs, he should have maximum compression (back feet close together, back relaxed and rounded, and head down).

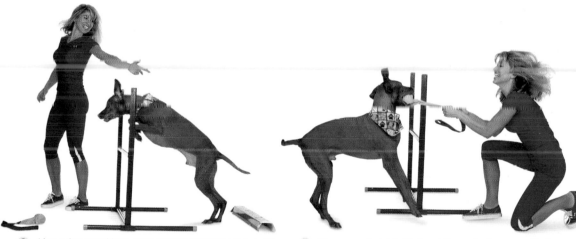

3 After a few repetitions, your dog will problem-solve on his own, and figure out how to jump efficiently. If your dog jumps over both jumps in one motion, move the jump bump back in 3 inch (8 cm) increments.

4 When your dog gets his toy at the end, play energetically with him as his reward.

TIP:

This is a problem-solving exercise, and is not intended to have a lot of repetitions. Repeat only three or four times in a session, with no more than three sessions per week.

EQUIPMENT:

Jump bumps are 4 to 8 inches (10 to 20 cm) wide and 40 inches (1 m) long, and can be made from plastic rain gutters. For small dogs (such as Shetland sheepdogs and Parson Russell terriers), set the jump bump 4 feet (1 m) in front of the jump. For medium size dogs (such as border collies), set it 5 feet (1.5 m) in front of the jump, and for large dogs set it 6 feet (2 m) in front of the jump.

BUILD ON IT:

Jumping Grid
page 108

Jumping Grid

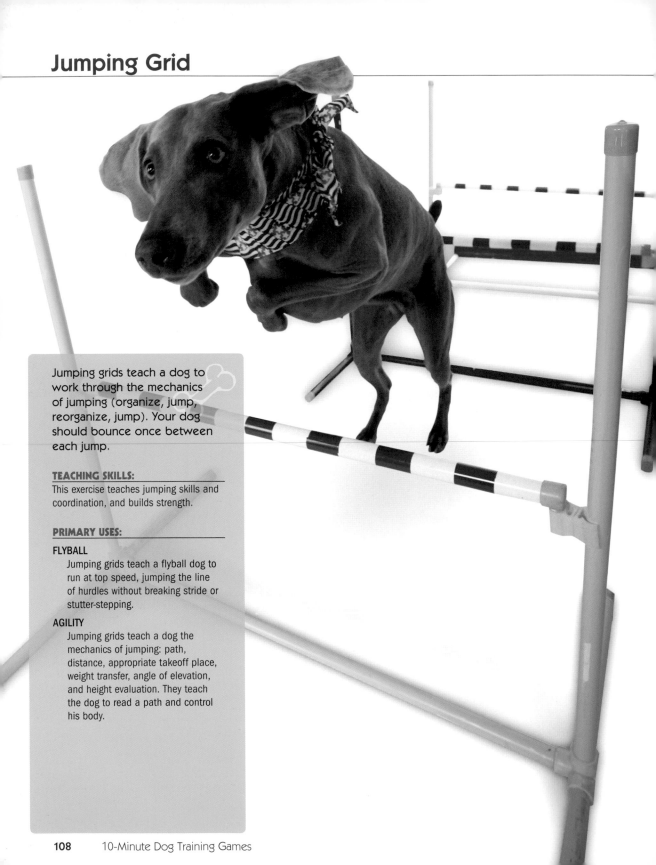

Jumping grids teach a dog to work through the mechanics of jumping (organize, jump, reorganize, jump). Your dog should bounce once between each jump.

TEACHING SKILLS:

This exercise teaches jumping skills and coordination, and builds strength.

PRIMARY USES:

FLYBALL

Jumping grids teach a flyball dog to run at top speed, jumping the line of hurdles without breaking stride or stutter-stepping.

AGILITY

Jumping grids teach a dog the mechanics of jumping: path, distance, appropriate takeoff place, weight transfer, angle of elevation, and height evaluation. They teach the dog to read a path and control his body.

TRY IT:

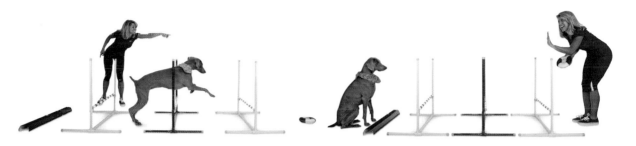

1 **Sending to target.** First, practice Stride Regulators (page 106). Next, set up three to five jumps in a straight line, equal distance apart, with a jump bump ahead of the first jump. Set your dog's toy (or a treat in a food dish) two stride lengths past the last jump. Stand with your dog behind the jump bump and send him to the target.

2 **Leading out.** For the next repetition, practice a leading-out exercise, which is used at agility competition start lines. Have your dog sit stay behind the jump bump and walk out to the end of the line.

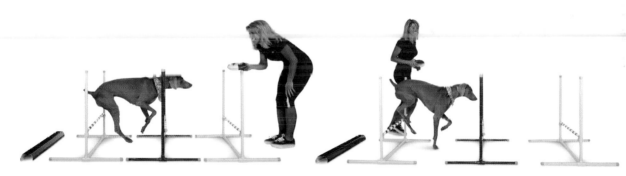

3 Release your dog to run toward you, taking the jumps along the way. Give him his reward from your hand when he gets to you.

4 **Motion.** In a motion exercise, your dog continues to take jumps even while you are running. Hold your dog's reward and run alongside your dog through the line of jumps.

TIP:	EQUIPMENT:	BUILD ON IT:
Excitable dogs may not be able to control themselves for the entire line of jumps, and their form may fall apart midway down the line. Perform just three repetitions of this exercise per session.	Set bar jumps in a straight line, at equal distance and equal height. For large dogs, space jumps 5 to 6 feet (1.5 to 1.8 m) apart at a height of 12 to 16 inches (30 to 40 cm). If your dog adds an extra stride between jumps instead of bouncing, reduce the spacing between the jumps.	Platform Jump *page 30* Cik & Cap Jump Wraps *page 110*

Cik & Cap Jump Wraps

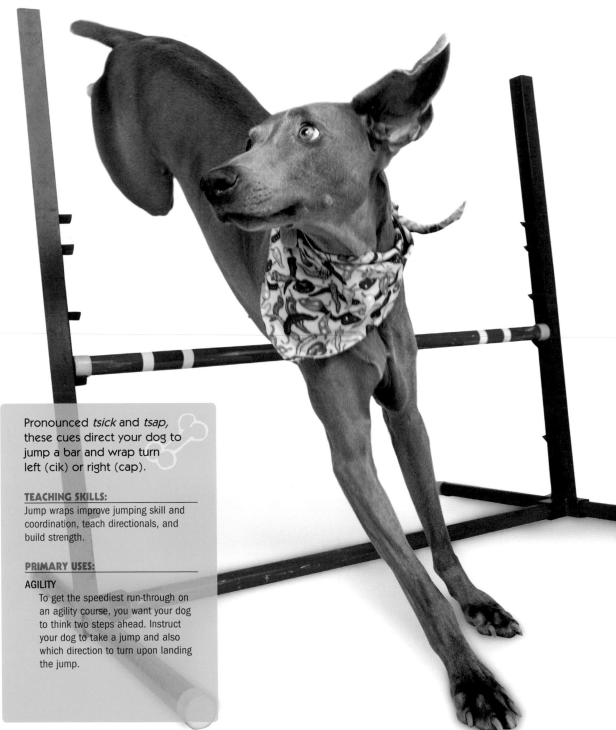

Pronounced *tsick* and *tsap*, these cues direct your dog to jump a bar and wrap turn left (cik) or right (cap).

TEACHING SKILLS:

Jump wraps improve jumping skill and coordination, teach directionals, and build strength.

PRIMARY USES:

AGILITY

To get the speediest run-through on an agility course, you want your dog to think two steps ahead. Instruct your dog to take a jump and also which direction to turn upon landing the jump.

TRY IT:

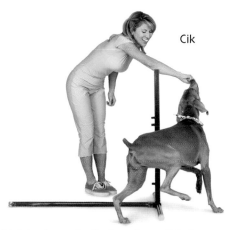

Cik

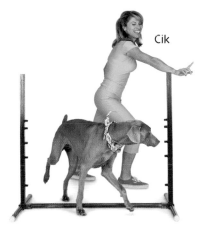

Cik

1 First, teach your dog Bar Jump (page 104). Set up only one upright of a bar jump. Lure your dog around the upright, using your right hand and the command "cik" for a counterclockwise turn. Give your dog the treat when he finishes the turn. Use your left hand and "cap" for clockwise circles.

2 Add the second upright. Stand a few feet behind the uprights. For a "cik," start with your dog on your right. Use your right arm to send him (as if you are pushing him), twist your right shoulder toward the jump, and take a step with your right foot toward the jump.

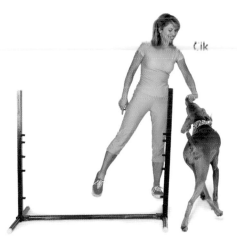

Cik

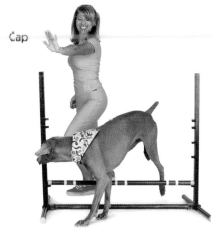

Cap

3 As your dog heads back to you, sidestep to your left and reward him with your left hand.

4 Set up the bar jump at a low height and try it again. In a "cap," push with your left hand and step with your left foot.

TIP:	**EQUIPMENT:**	**BUILD ON IT:**
Work on both "cik" and "cap" at the same time, alternating. Remember to cue your dog BEFORE he takes the jump, as once he is in the air he has already committed to his landing point.	Construct a bar jump from PVC plastic pipes and connectors. Jump cups to snap onto the poles and allow the bar to roll off, should your dog accidentally knock it.	Jumping Figure-8s *page 112* Barrel Racing *page 142*

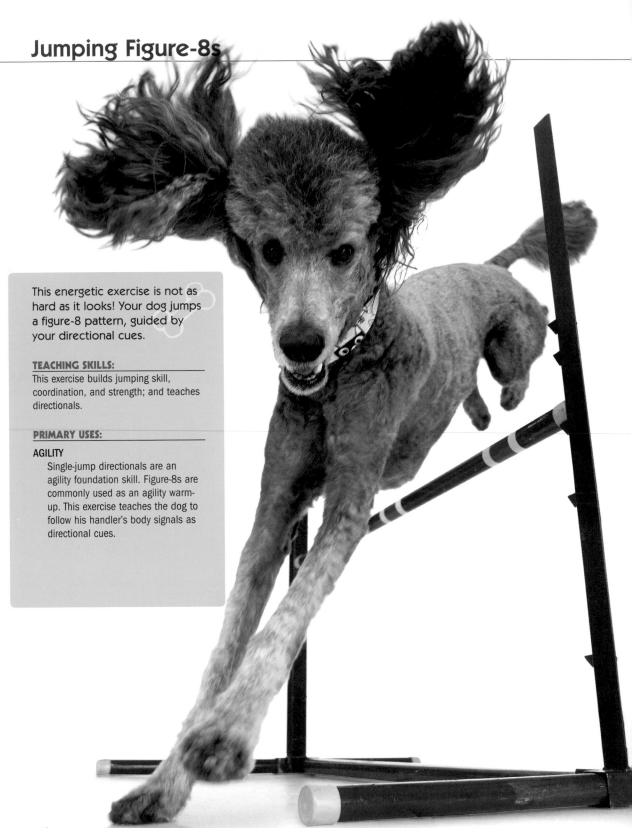

Jumping Figure-8s

This energetic exercise is not as hard as it looks! Your dog jumps a figure-8 pattern, guided by your directional cues.

TEACHING SKILLS:

This exercise builds jumping skill, coordination, and strength; and teaches directionals.

PRIMARY USES:

AGILITY

Single-jump directionals are an agility foundation skill. Figure-8s are commonly used as an agility warm-up. This exercise teaches the dog to follow his handler's body signals as directional cues.

TRY IT:

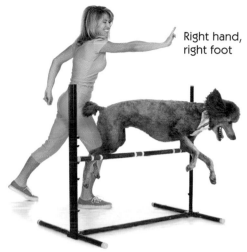

Right hand,
right foot

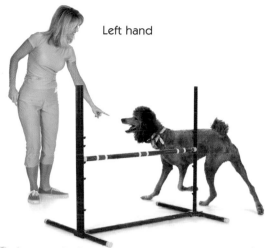

Left hand

1 First, teach your dog Cick & Cap Jump Wraps (page 110). Stand behind the jump with your dog on your right. Say, "Hup!" (or "Cik!") and push your right hand toward the left upright. Step with your right foot toward the left upright.

2 Once your dog is committed to the jump, realign your feet together at the center. Use a pointed finger on your left hand to draw your dog back to your left side.

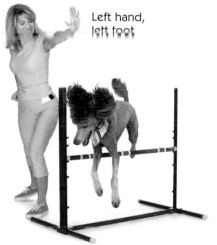

Left hand,
left foot

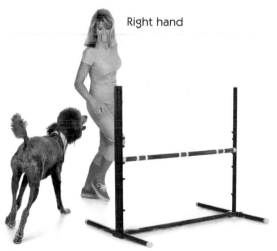

Right hand

3 Say, "Hup!" (or "Cap!") and push your left hand toward the right upright. Step with your left foot toward the right upright.

4 Once your dog has committed to the jump, realign your feet and use your right-hand pointed finger to draw your dog back to your right side.

TIP:

Practice this dance on your own before involving your dog. A skilled handler can guide a new dog through this exercise in their first session.

EQUIPMENT:

Construct a bar jump from PVC plastic pipes and connectors. Jump cups snap onto the poles and allow the bar to fall off, should your dog accidentally knock it.

BUILD ON IT:

Barrel Racing
page 142

Laser Light

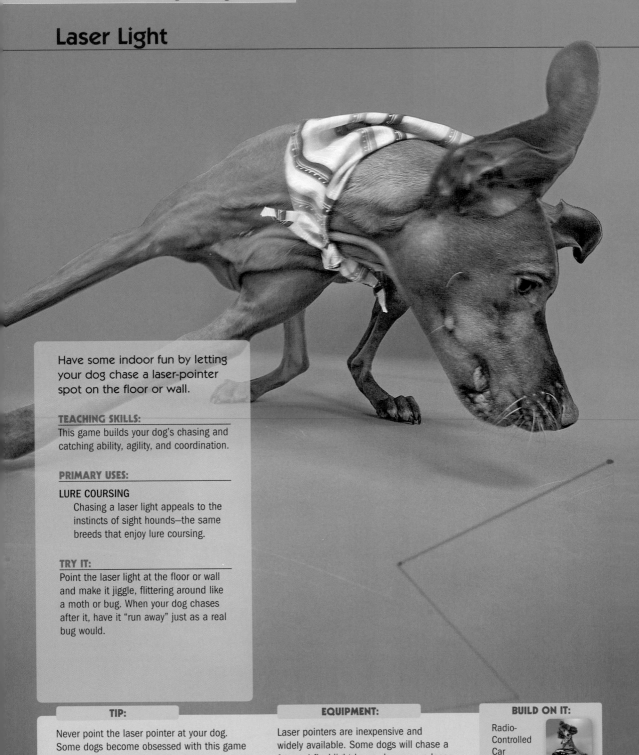

Have some indoor fun by letting your dog chase a laser-pointer spot on the floor or wall.

TEACHING SKILLS:

This game builds your dog's chasing and catching ability, agility, and coordination.

PRIMARY USES:

LURE COURSING

Chasing a laser light appeals to the instincts of sight hounds—the same breeds that enjoy lure coursing.

TRY IT:

Point the laser light at the floor or wall and make it jiggle, flittering around like a moth or bug. When your dog chases after it, have it "run away" just as a real bug would.

TIP:

Never point the laser pointer at your dog. Some dogs become obsessed with this game to the point of having anxiety. So long as your dog enjoys it in moderation, it is fine.

EQUIPMENT:

Laser pointers are inexpensive and widely available. Some dogs will chase a focused flashlight beam; however, a laser light tends to be more enticing.

BUILD ON IT:

Radio-Controlled Car
page 115

Radio-Controlled Car

RC cars promise all the fun of chasing a skittering prey animal!

TEACHING SKILLS:

This game builds your dog's chasing and catching ability, as well as his agility and coordination.

PRIMARY USES:

LURE COURSING

In lure coursing, a dog chases a fur pelt or plastic bag that is pulled on a line. Chasing an RC car is a similar game, and even allows you finer control of the chase object.

TRY IT:

Take care not to scare your dog with the toy. Initially, drive it far away from your dog. It will be more fun for your dog if the car runs away from him like a real prey animal, rather than toward him. Have the car stop, and when your dog comes forward to investigate it . . . have it run away!

TIP:

Dogs either love this game or they don't. Give it a try and see if it entices your dog!

EQUIPMENT:

Attaching some ribbons or furry strips to the back of the toy can initially help entice your dog to chase it.

BUILD ON IT:

Lunge Whip
page 116

Lunge Whip

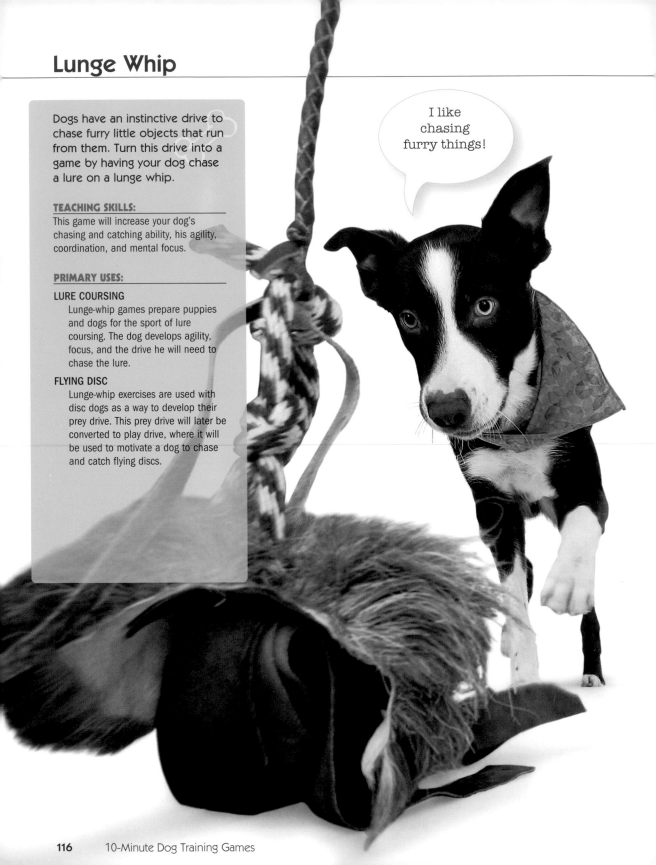

Dogs have an instinctive drive to chase furry little objects that run from them. Turn this drive into a game by having your dog chase a lure on a lunge whip.

TEACHING SKILLS:

This game will increase your dog's chasing and catching ability, his agility, coordination, and mental focus.

PRIMARY USES:

LURE COURSING

Lunge-whip games prepare puppies and dogs for the sport of lure coursing. The dog develops agility, focus, and the drive he will need to chase the lure.

FLYING DISC

Lunge-whip exercises are used with disc dogs as a way to develop their prey drive. This prey drive will later be converted to play drive, where it will be used to motivate a dog to chase and catch flying discs.

I like chasing furry things!

TRY IT:

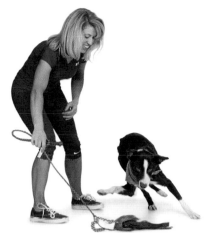

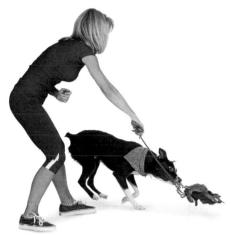

1 Build your dog's interest in the lunge whip by whisking it on the ground in an erratic fashion—always skittering AWAY from your dog. If your dog is hesitant, let the toy rest on the ground and then skitter away in fear if your dog approaches.

2 Your toy should imitate a real prey animal that doesn't want to be caught. Keep the toy just out of your dog's reach, building prey drive to the maximum.

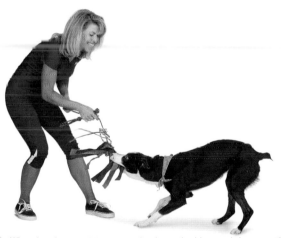

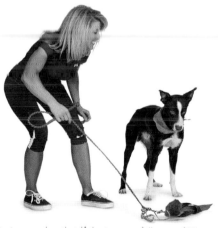

3 When he chases with great enthusiasm, let him catch it. Play a little tug once your dog catches it, moving the toy smoothly side to side (not a backward/forward tug), with an occasional careful jerk.

4 Just remember that if the toy ever falls out of his mouth, it goes back to being live prey that tries to run away from him again!

TIP:	EQUIPMENT:	BUILD ON IT:

TIP:
Different dogs will have more or less prey-drive instinct and interest in this game. For dogs who are reluctant at first, try incorporating a squeaker or food pocket into the lure to make it more enticing.

EQUIPMENT:
A lunge whip (also called longe whip or lure pole) can be purchased at a farm store. Make your own with a flexible lash of about 5 feet (1.5 m). On the end, affix a lure made from animal pelt, leather or fleece strips, or a plastic bag.

BUILD ON IT:
Tug
page 124

Disc Rollers

Rollers are great fun (and exercise) for your dog. Your dog learns to seize the disc while it is rolling, without the added difficulty of catching it in the air.

TEACHING SKILLS:
Disc rollers teach chasing and catching skills and coordination.

PRIMARY USES:

FLYING DISC
Disc rollers are the first step in teaching a dog to catch a flying disc.

LURE COURSING
Chasing a rolling disc is the same skill as chasing an artificial lure. Rollers will give you a variation in your training options.

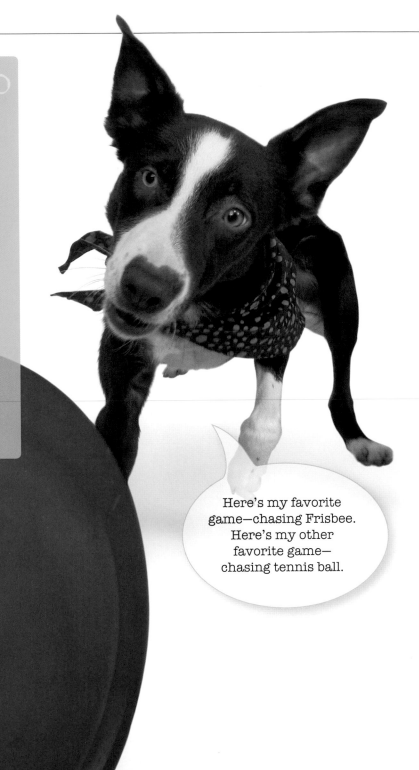

Here's my favorite game—chasing Frisbee. Here's my other favorite game—chasing tennis ball.

TRY IT:

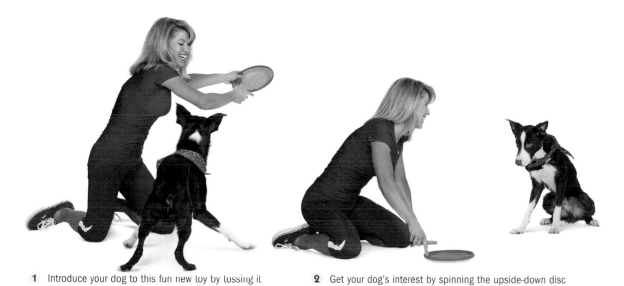

1 Introduce your dog to this fun new toy by tossing it playfully or playing keep away or tug with it.

2 Get your dog's interest by spinning the upside-down disc in circles.

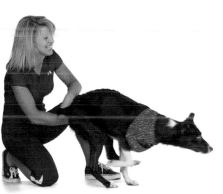

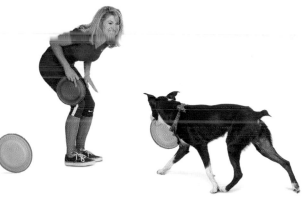

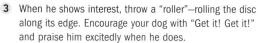

3 When he shows interest, throw a "roller"—rolling the disc along its edge. Encourage your dog with "Get it! Get it!" and praise him excitedly when he does.

4 Encourage him to bring the disc back to you by clapping your hands and calling to him. Have a second disc, and when he comes, immediately throw the new disc. If he does not come, do not chase him, but rather turn your back and ignore him.

TIP:	**EQUIPMENT:**	**BUILD ON IT:**
If your dog is not interested in the disc, increase its value by turning it upside down and using it as your dog's feeding dish. He will come to associate the sight and smell of it with his dinner.	Hard plastic toy discs could injure your dog's mouth and teeth. Use only discs specifically designed for a dog, such as a soft plastic, flexible rubber, or canvas disc.	Disc Catch *page 120*

Disc Catch

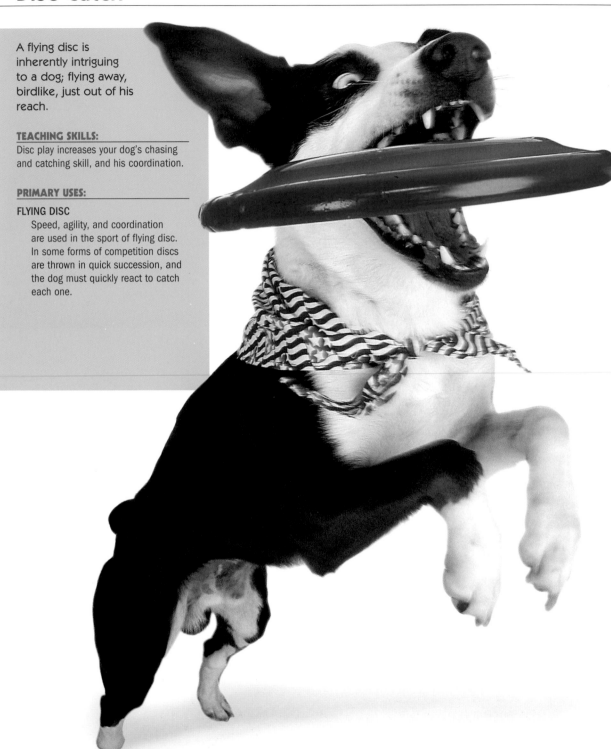

A flying disc is inherently intriguing to a dog; flying away, birdlike, just out of his reach.

TEACHING SKILLS:
Disc play increases your dog's chasing and catching skill, and his coordination.

PRIMARY USES:

FLYING DISC
Speed, agility, and coordination are used in the sport of flying disc. In some forms of competition discs are thrown in quick succession, and the dog must quickly react to catch each one.

TRY IT:

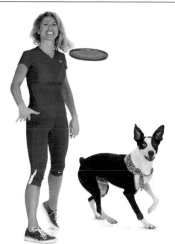

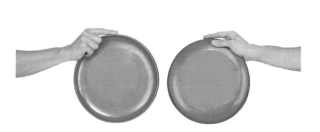

1 First, work with your dog on Disc Rollers (page 118). Train on a soft surface that has good traction (lush grass is ideal). Hold the disc parallel to the ground, with your fingers curled under the inside edge, your index finger slightly extended.

2 Start with your dog near you and throw the disc so it is flying AWAY from your dog and not toward him. With your shoulders perpendicular to your target, pull the disc across your body. Snap your wrist just before you release the disc.

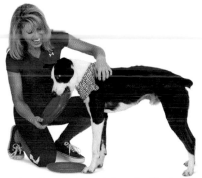

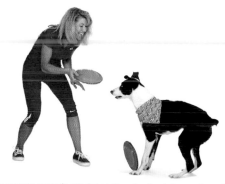

3 If your dog attempts to catch it, praise him lavishly and throw another disc. If he simply watches it fall to the ground, go back to building drive and desire with disc rollers.

4 Encourage your dog to bring the disc back to you by using two identical discs and enthusiastically presenting the second disc while showing no interest in the disc your dog is holding. Throw the second disc the moment the first one is dropped, so your dog thinks that he is causing you to throw the second disc.

TIP:

Dogs should jump in such a way that they land with four paws on the ground, rather than vertically (which could stress their spine and knees). There is considerable human skill required in throwing a disc, which is why you should be practicing three times as many throws as your dog practices catches.

EQUIPMENT:

Hard plastic toy discs could injure your dog's mouth and teeth. Use discs specifically designed for a dog, such as a soft plastic, flexible rubber, or canvas discs.

BUILD ON IT:

Fetch
page 144

Volleyball
page 154

Scootering

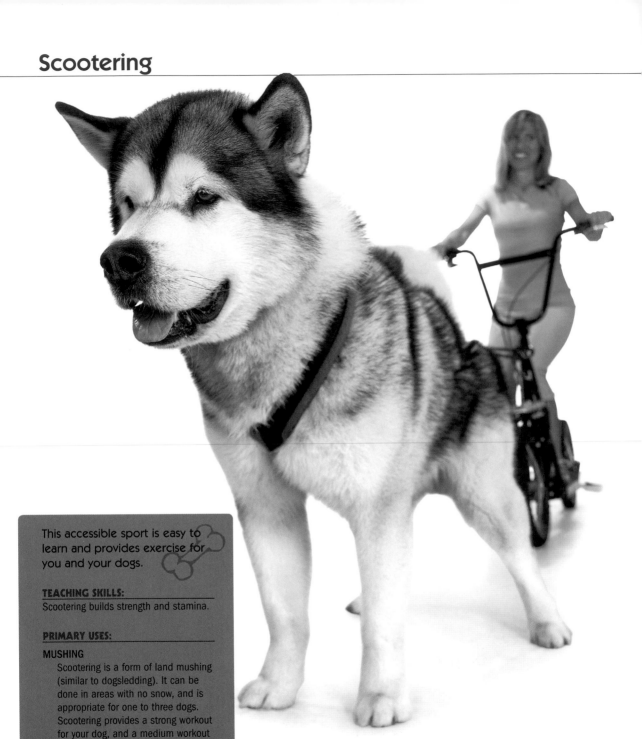

This accessible sport is easy to learn and provides exercise for you and your dogs.

TEACHING SKILLS:
Scootering builds strength and stamina.

PRIMARY USES:

MUSHING
Scootering is a form of land mushing (similar to dogsledding). It can be done in areas with no snow, and is appropriate for one to three dogs. Scootering provides a strong workout for your dog, and a medium workout for yourself.

TRY IT:

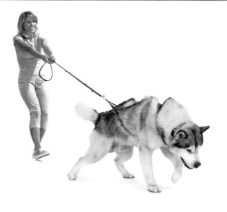

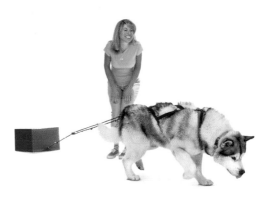

1 Attach a tugline to the back ring of your dog's harness. Set out your dog's food dish with a few treats in it. Tell him enthusiastically to "Hike!" This cue word will come to mean that he should pull.

2 Attach the tugline to a box and try it again. The sound of the box moving may startle your dog, so stay close and give him lots of encouragement. Avoid going in front of your dog, as on a scooter your position will be behind him.

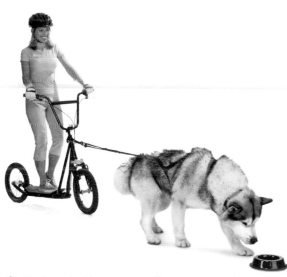

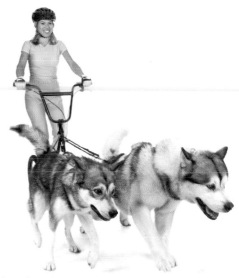

3 Finally, try it with your scooter. Keep your eye on the tugline so that it does not go slack and under your wheel.

4 Up to three dogs can run comfortably with a scooter. Dogs run best in cool temperatures and in wilderness environments which are new and exciting to them.

TIP:	EQUIPMENT:	BUILD ON IT:

A dog will be more enthusiastic to run when he is competing against other dogs. Get some friends and their dogs together and go scootering as a group.

Specially-made dog scooters have off-road tires and a solid construction. The dog wears a mushing harness that is attached to the scooter by a tugline with sections of bungee. A coupler and neckline are used with a second dog. Wear a helmet, gloves, sunglasses or goggles, and appropriate shoes. Bring water, first aid, and a cellphone or GPS.

Assisted Upright Walking *page 126*

Tug

Many dogs really enjoy tugging games with their owner. This high-energy game has become popular among dog trainers as a way of rewarding a dog.

TEACHING SKILLS:

This game builds your dog's strength.

PRIMARY USES:

DOG SPORTS MOTIVATOR
Using a tug toy as a reward has become widely popular in high-energy dog sports such as agility, flyball, dock diving, Schutzhund, and obedience. Once the dog gets to really like the game of tug, we can use that as a reward for a good effort in a dog sport.

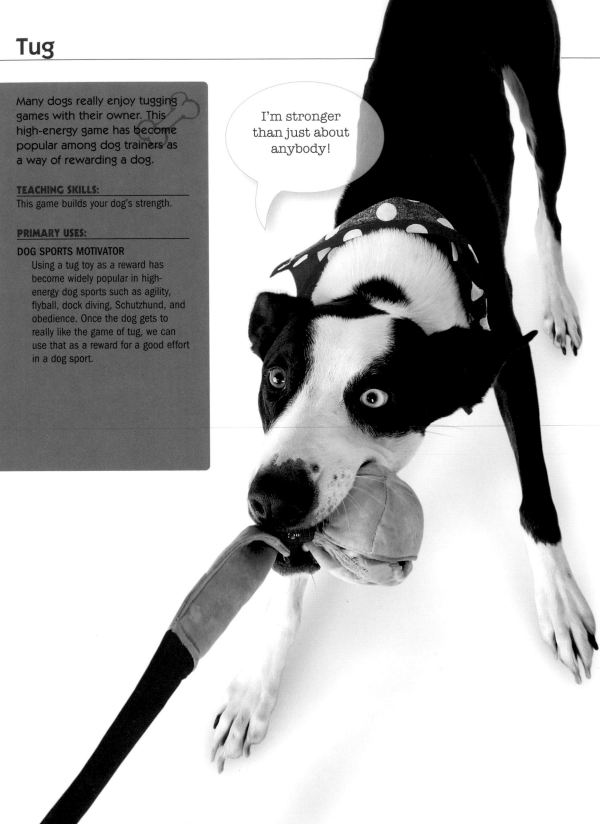

I'm stronger than just about anybody!

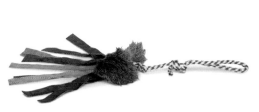

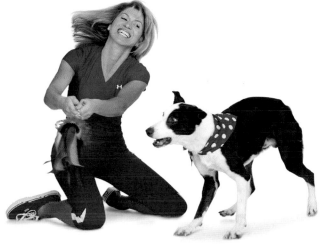

1 Choose a tug toy that is long and whippy, with fur, fleece, or leather hanging pieces. Squeakers or food pockets will be extra enticing.

2 Play with the toy, always moving it away from your dog so he has to chase it. Toss it in the air and catch it, or toss it across the yard and race him toward it.

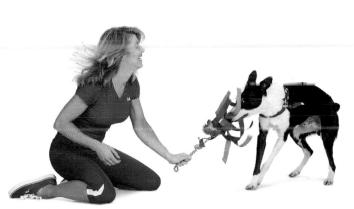

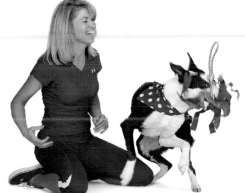

3 Once your dog is excited, let him catch the toy and say, "Tug!" Move the toy smoothly side to side (not a backward/forward tug), with an occasional, careful jerk.

4 After a few seconds of tugging, let your dog pull the toy from your hands as his reward. If your dog is reluctant to tug, let go of the toy as soon as he bites it and give him lots of praise.

TIP:

Dogs who aren't interested in tugging at first may respond to food tug toys—mesh tubes that can be stuffed with mushy food.

EQUIPMENT:

Start with a toy that is long and whippy and easy to manipulate, and of a thin, easy-to-grab material. Good drive-building toys are made from fleece, fur, or leather. They have hanging pieces (such as octopus shapes). The toys may come with squeakers or food pouches, which can help to entice reluctant dogs.

BUILD ON IT:

Logic Test
page 38

Fishing with a Rope
page 40

Assisted Upright Walking

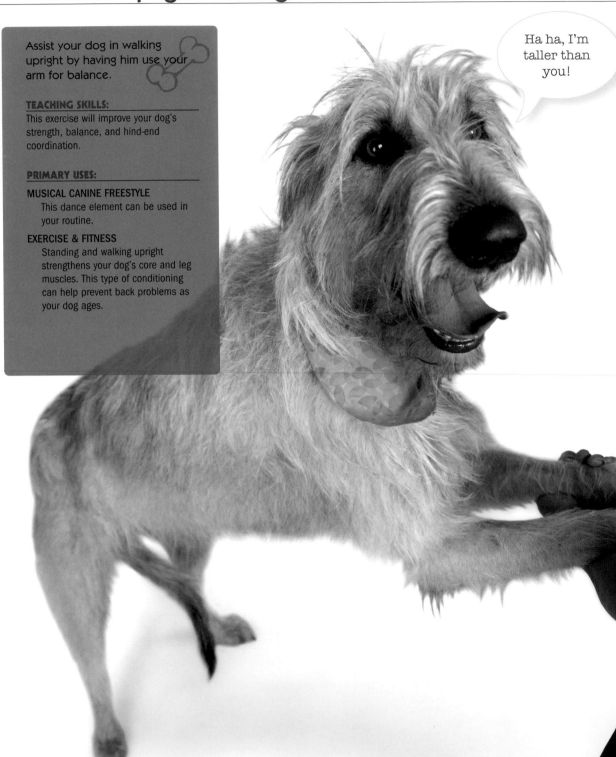

Assist your dog in walking upright by having him use your arm for balance.

TEACHING SKILLS:

This exercise will improve your dog's strength, balance, and hind-end coordination.

PRIMARY USES:

MUSICAL CANINE FREESTYLE

This dance element can be used in your routine.

EXERCISE & FITNESS

Standing and walking upright strengthens your dog's core and leg muscles. This type of conditioning can help prevent back problems as your dog ages.

Ha ha, I'm taller than you!

TRY IT:

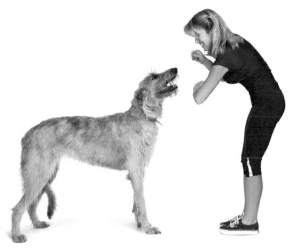

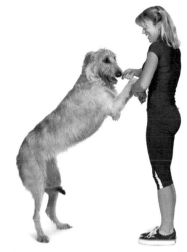

1 Hold your arm in front of your chest, which is your strongest position. Use a treat in your other hand to lure your dog to place his front paws onto your arm. If your dog is comfortable with you doing so, you can also lift his paws onto your arm.

2 Make this a rewarding place for your dog by letting him nibble treats from your hand (it will be helpful to start with a handful of treats).

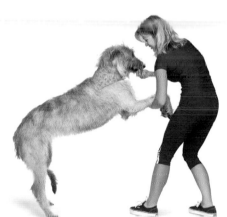

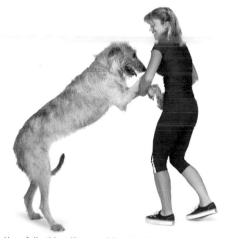

3 After a while, take a small step backward and pull the treat slightly away from your dog, so that he has to reach forward for it.

4 Hopefully this will cause him to take a step toward you. Now he's walking!

TIP:

This exercise takes strength and may be tiring for your dog. If he continually jumps down from your arm, it may be that he is becoming tired. Once dogs get the hang of this, they can walk with you all the way across the room!

BUILD ON IT:

Peanut Roll
page 98

Sit High
page 128

Sit High

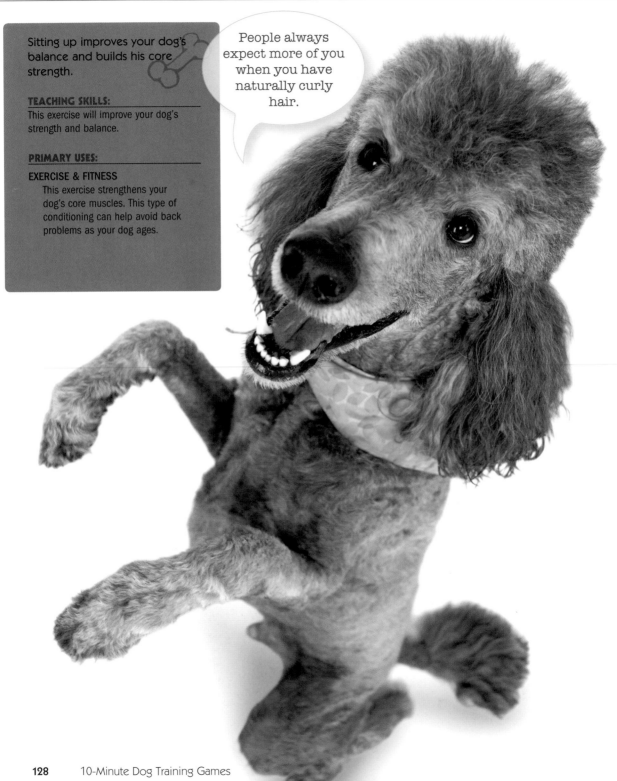

Sitting up improves your dog's balance and builds his core strength.

TEACHING SKILLS:
This exercise will improve your dog's strength and balance.

PRIMARY USES:

EXERCISE & FITNESS
This exercise strengthens your dog's core muscles. This type of conditioning can help avoid back problems as your dog ages.

People always expect more of you when you have naturally curly hair.

TRY IT:

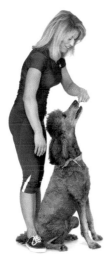

1 Have your dog sit. Stand directly behind him, with your heels together and your toes pointed apart. Hold a treat in front of his nose to keep his attention.

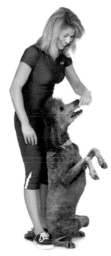

2 Use your treat to slowly guide his head back and straight up.

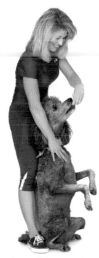

3 Steady his chest with your other hand and allow him to nibble treats while in this position.

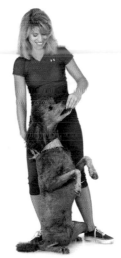

4 Move one leg away so that your dog is leaning against only one of your legs. Support the back of his neck with your hand. Your dog will need more strength to balance in this position.

TIP:

Some dogs will be able to do this exercise easily, while others (often larger dogs) may have a much harder time finding their balance. If your dog is jumping at the treat, move it more slowly. If your dog stands up on his hind legs, keep your hand lower and say, "Sit." Hold the treat at his face height.

BUILD ON IT:

Assisted Upright Walking
page 126

Follow Pointed Finger

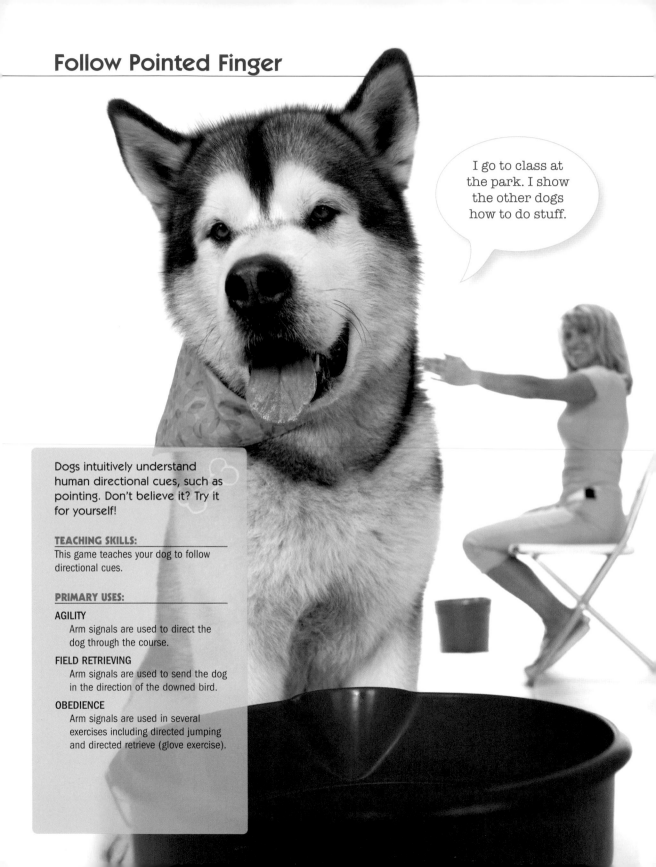

I go to class at the park. I show the other dogs how to do stuff.

Dogs intuitively understand human directional cues, such as pointing. Don't believe it? Try it for yourself!

TEACHING SKILLS:
This game teaches your dog to follow directional cues.

PRIMARY USES:

AGILITY
Arm signals are used to direct the dog through the course.

FIELD RETRIEVING
Arm signals are used to send the dog in the direction of the downed bird.

OBEDIENCE
Arm signals are used in several exercises including directed jumping and directed retrieve (glove exercise).

TRY IT:

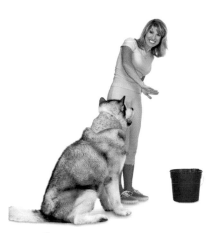
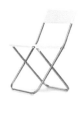
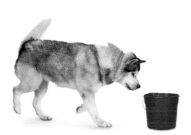
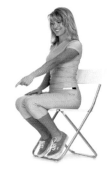

1 Place a treat in a bucket but don't let your dog know that it is there. Put him in a sit-stay.

2 Point to the bucket and tell your dog, "Go!" Let him find and eat the treat. Repeat this exercise as many times as it takes until your dog goes quickly and directly to the bucket.

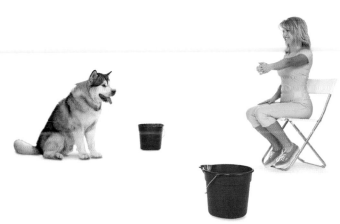
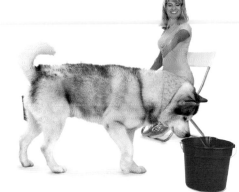

3 Set out two buckets, one on either side of you. Only one bucket will have a treat. Point to the loaded bucket and cue, "Go!"

4 If your dog heads to the wrong bucket, stop him and start the game again. Do not allow him to follow through. If he goes to the correct bucket, he gets the treat!

TIP:	EQUIPMENT:	BUILD ON IT:

Your dog may surprise you and do better than you think! If your dog is having trouble holding his sit-stay, have a friend hold your dog. The friend should say and do as little as possible, to avoid influencing your dog.

Use two identical buckets or boxes large enough that your dog can easily insert his head and retrieve the treat.

Directional Casting
page 138

Target Mat

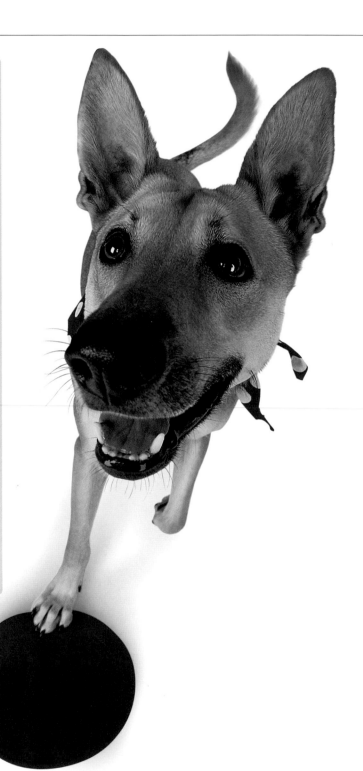

Your dog runs to step on a specific mark.

TEACHING SKILLS:
This game teaches going to a mark and directional cues.

PRIMARY USES:

ANIMAL ACTOR
The first behavior an animal actor learns is to "go to a mark" on stage. A very small target mat is used for the mark.

MUSICAL CANINE FREESTYLE
One of the more difficult skills in freestyle is teaching a dog to run away from the handler to a specific spot. Target mats, or touch pads, are used to teach this skill.

AGILITY
A target mat is placed at the base of a contact obstacle (such as an A-frame) to teach the dog to stop at the base of the obstacle.

OBEDIENCE
Target mats are used to train the "go out" exercise, where the dog runs in a straight line away from the handler.

TRY IT:

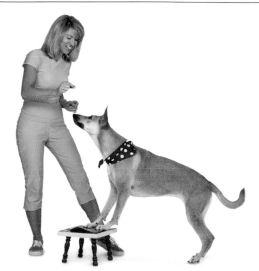

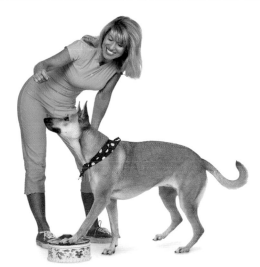

1 Affix your target mat to the top of a short stool. Hold a treat to your dog's nose, and move it slowly above the stool. As soon as your dog steps on the stool, say, "Good!" and give him the treat.

2 Next, affix the target mat to a slightly smaller and shorter object, such as an upside-down dog bowl. Say, "Target!" and lure him to step on it. Always give your dog his reward while his paws are on the mat and not after they've come off.

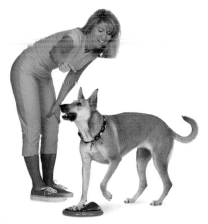

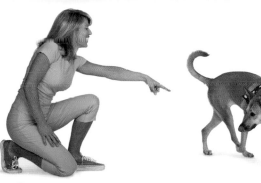

3 Affix the target mat to a shorter object, such as a flying disc. If at any point your dog seems confused, go back to a previous step.

4 Finally, lay the target mat directly on the floor. By this point you should be able to send your dog to the target instead of directly luring him.

TIP:

While you may be tempted to skip a few steps and rush to put the target mat on the ground, you will find quicker success by progressing through incremental height levels of the target. The levels go quickly, and you may be able to progress through them with a few repetitions of each.

EQUIPMENT:

Make your own target mat from a metal jar lid, a carpet sample, a drink coaster, or whatever you wish. Very flat items or metal items work best, as your dog won't be tempted to pick them up in his mouth.

BUILD ON IT:

Doggie Doorbell
page 134

Doggie Doorbell

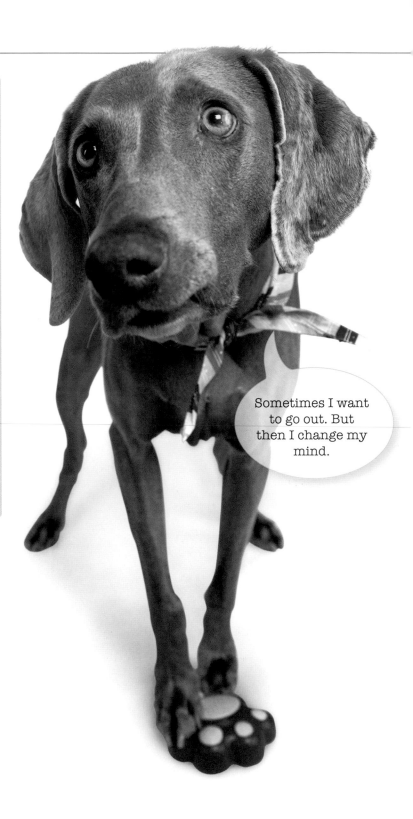

Tired of your dog scratching at the door? Teach him to step on an electronic doggie doorbell instead. How convenient!

TEACHING SKILLS:
This game improves communication and coordination and teaches going to a mark.

PRIMARY USES:

HOUSE-TRAINING
Doggie doorbells can be used on either side of the door, for when your dog wants to go out or for when he wants to come inside the house. This behavior is especially helpful during potty training.

SERVICE DOG
Service dogs can be trained to press an emergency button on the telephone or press a tap light to turn it on.

Sometimes I want to go out. But then I change my mind.

TRY IT:

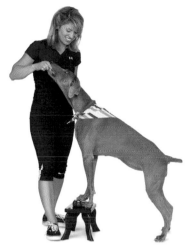

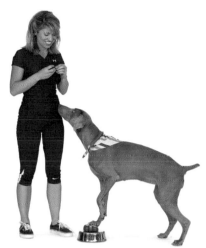

1 Securely tape your doggie doorbell to a short stool. Use a treat to lure your dog to step onto the stool. When he does, say, "Good!" and give him the treat. If he happens to step on the doorbell itself and make it chime, give him three treats and excited praise!

2 Next, tape the doggie doorbell to a smaller object, such as an upside-down dog bowl. Stand opposite from your dog, with the doorbell between you. Say, "Doorbell!" and try to get him to step on it. Give him a treat if he touches the doorbell (even if it doesn't actually chime).

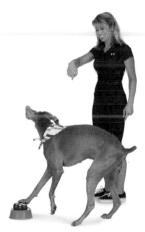

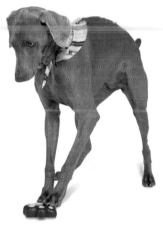

3 Tape the doggie doorbell to an even smaller object. With such a small object, your dog will be making the doorbell chime almost every time he steps on it. Reward him every time you hear the chime.

4 Finally, affix the doorbell directly to the floor. Your dog may try to scratch at the doorbell, so it will need to be secured to the floor.

TIP:	EQUIPMENT:	BUILD ON IT:

Once your dog gets the hang of stepping on the doorbell, have him step on it before opening the door for him. He'll soon get the idea!

Electronic doggie doorbells are battery operated and composed of the button component that your dog steps on, and a small, wireless speaker. The speaker can be placed up to about 40 feet (12 m) from the button.

Ring a Bell to Go Out *page 152*

Pedestal

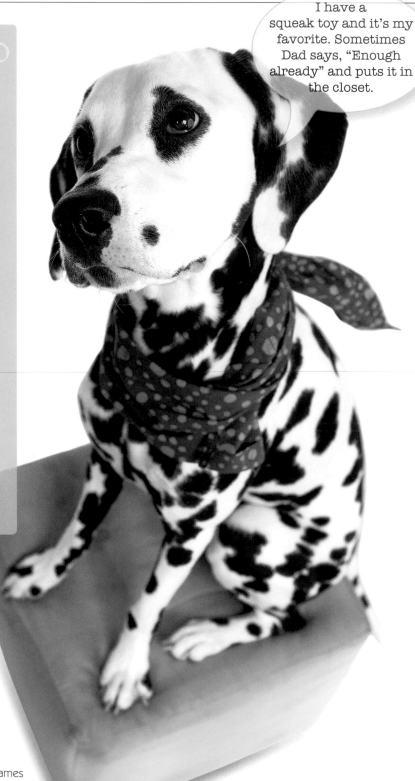

Dogs are naturally height-seekers and quickly learn to enjoy their spot on a pedestal.

TEACHING SKILLS:

This game teaches your dog self control and staying on a mark.

PRIMARY USES:

AGILITY

The pedestal is similar to the "pause table" obstacle in the sport of agility.

MANNERS & SELF-CONTROL

Pedestal training (also called "spot training") means that the dog goes to and remains on his spot (which can be simply his dog bed). Spot training is used during dinnertime or when visitors arrive as a way to keep your dog still and in control. It is easiest to teach this skill first with a raised pedestal rather than with a dog bed, because dogs tend to try to creep out of a lower spot.

SEARCH AND RESCUE

A SAR dog must demonstrate the ability to jump at least 2¹/₂ feet (76 cm) up onto a pedestal.

I have a squeak toy and it's my favorite. Sometimes Dad says, "Enough already" and puts it in the closet.

TRY IT:

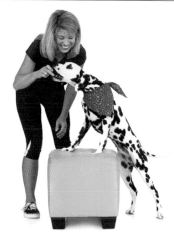

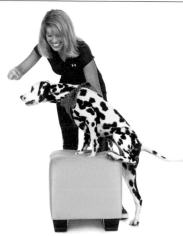

1 Get your dog interested in a treat and slowly lift it up over the pedestal. Your dog will put his paws on the pedestal, trying to reach the treat. When he does, let him nibble the treat in your hand.

2 Now say, "Step up" and continue to draw the treat farther across the pedestal, so that your dog has to climb on top to reach it. If your dog keeps circling the pedestal, give him an occasional treat for just putting his front paws up so that he doesn't become discouraged and walk away.

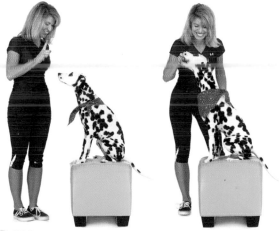

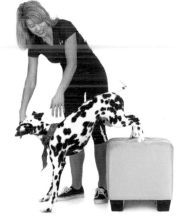

3 While your dog is on the pedestal, tell him to "stay" and keep giving him praise and treats while he remains up there. If he knows he will get occasional, random treats, he will be motivated to stay on his pedestal for longer and longer periods of time.

4 Your dog should stay on his pedestal until given the release word, "off." If he comes off prematurely, have him get back on (try first to get him on without a treat, but use a treat if you must.)

TIP:	EQUIPMENT:	BUILD ON IT:
A key training strategy is to reward your dog when he gets ON the pedestal, but to never reward him for getting OFF the pedestal (even if you told him to get off).	A pedestal should be raised and sturdy and should have a nonslip surface. Common pedestals are an upside-down horse water bucket, a raised dog bed, the top half of a plastic dog crate, a plyometric box, and an agility pause table.	Platform Jump *page 30* Directional Casting *page 138*

Directional Casting

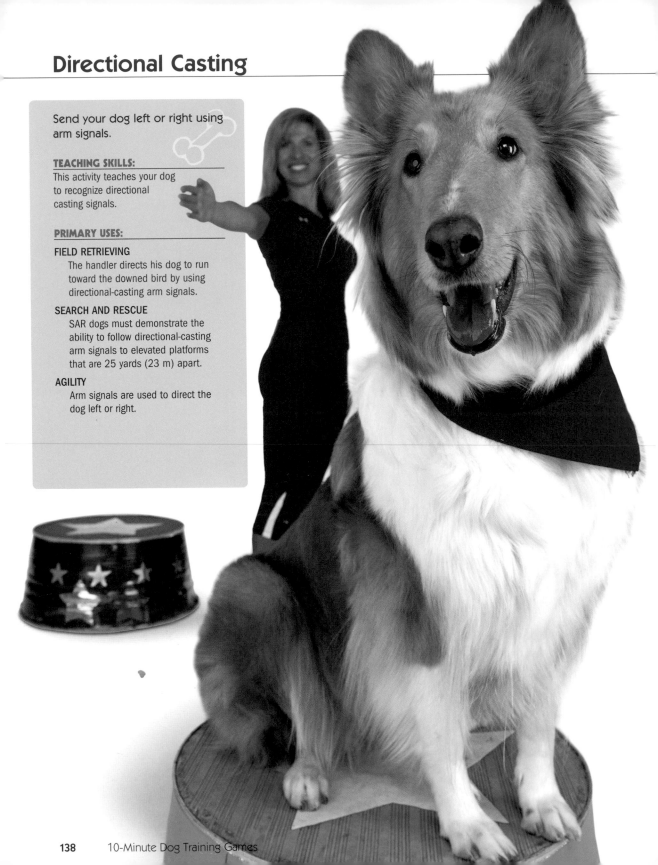

Send your dog left or right using arm signals.

TEACHING SKILLS:

This activity teaches your dog to recognize directional casting signals.

PRIMARY USES:

FIELD RETRIEVING
The handler directs his dog to run toward the downed bird by using directional-casting arm signals.

SEARCH AND RESCUE
SAR dogs must demonstrate the ability to follow directional-casting arm signals to elevated platforms that are 25 yards (23 m) apart.

AGILITY
Arm signals are used to direct the dog left or right.

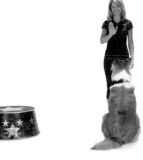
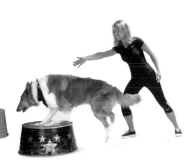

1 First, teach your dog to get on a Pedestal (page 136). Put your dog in a sit-stay, with a platform on either side of him and slightly forward of where he is sitting (as your dog will naturally want to move forward, toward you, in addition to going left or right).

2 Move slowly and deliberately. Extend your arm first and then say, "Step up" and lunge toward one platform. Be sure to give the arm signal a second before the lunge and verbal cue.

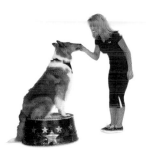

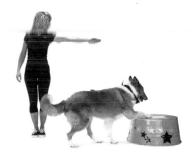

3 Walk forward and reward your dog while he is still on the platform. After a few seconds say, "Off," bring your dog back to the center, and try casting your dog to the other platform.

4 As your dog improves, you will no longer need to lunge toward the platform, and your dog will go simply based on your arm signal. If your dog heads to the wrong platform, stop him with your voice before he gets there. Set him back in the center and try again.

TIP:
Start with the platforms fairly close together and build up distance. After your dog has mastered left and right casting, add two more platforms and teach him to "come" and "go."

EQUIPMENT:
Use two identical raised platforms. Wooden platforms raised about 8 inches (20 cm) off the ground are commonly used in retrieving training.

BUILD ON IT:
Hand Signals
page 140

Hand Signals

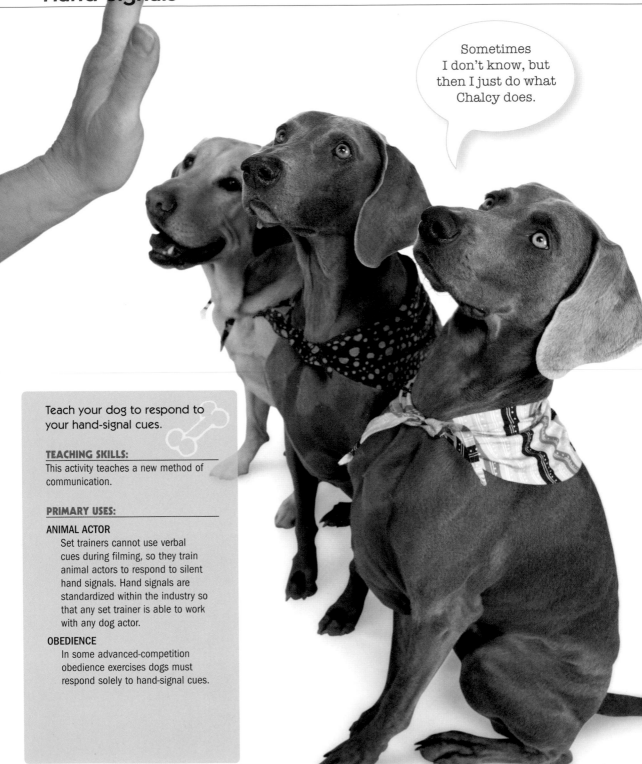

Sometimes I don't know, but then I just do what Chalcy does.

Teach your dog to respond to your hand-signal cues.

TEACHING SKILLS:

This activity teaches a new method of communication.

PRIMARY USES:

ANIMAL ACTOR

Set trainers cannot use verbal cues during filming, so they train animal actors to respond to silent hand signals. Hand signals are standardized within the industry so that any set trainer is able to work with any dog actor.

OBEDIENCE

In some advanced-competition obedience exercises dogs must respond solely to hand-signal cues.

TRY IT:

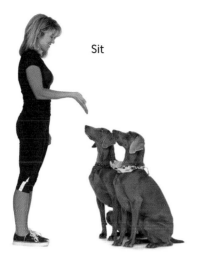

Sit

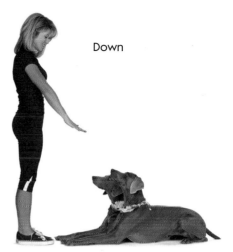

Down

1 Hand signals are derived from the luring motion we made when initially teaching the behavior. The "sit" hand signal looks like the motion of luring the dog's head up.

2 Start with a behavior that your dog already knows. Do the hand signal, wait one second, and then say your verbal cue. Reward your dog for doing the behavior.

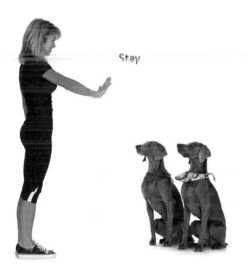

Stay

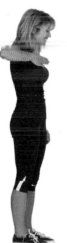

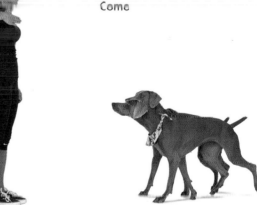

Come

3 Your dog wants her treat as quickly as possible. She will learn that your hand signal is always followed by your verbal cue. She will learn to perform the behavior already at your hand signal in order to get her treat more quickly.

4 Hold your hand and arm rigid and make your movements clean and precise.

TIP:

Dogs respond extremely well to hand signals. In fact, once your dog understands a hand signal, she will respond to your signal more readily than your verbal cue. If, for example, you say, "Sit" but give the hand signal for "down," your dog will probably lie down.

BUILD ON IT:

Directional Casting
page 138

Barrel Racing

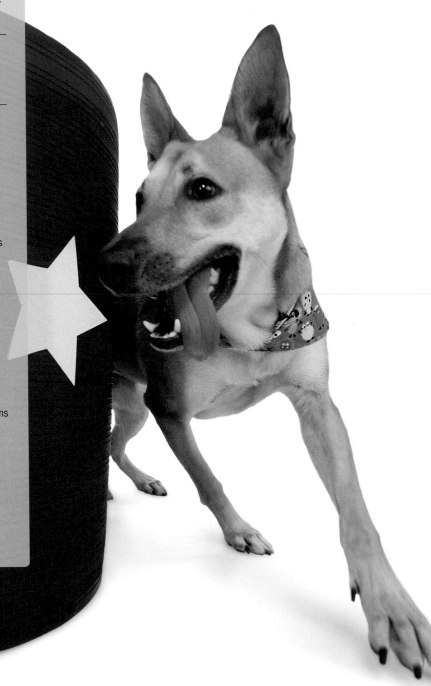

Originally an equestrian event, dogs compete for time running a course around several barrels.

TEACHING SKILLS:
This active game improves your dog's agility and teaches a "go around" directional cue.

PRIMARY USES:

BARREL-RACING COMPETITION
Barrel racing originated at rodeos, where horses race a cloverleaf pattern around three barrels. Dogs now compete in this sport as well. The handler stands behind the starting line and directs his dog around each barrel.

HERDING
When herding sheep, the dog circles around a group of sheep, gathering them in a tight group. Barrel racing is an introduction to this circling behavior.

AGILITY
The agility "forward send" cues the dog to run away from you and over an obstacle. Barrel racing is a type of forward send.

MUSICAL CANINE FREESTYLE
The "go-around" is a dancing foundation skill in which the dog runs away from his handler and circles a prop. Barrel racing is a go-around.

TRY IT:

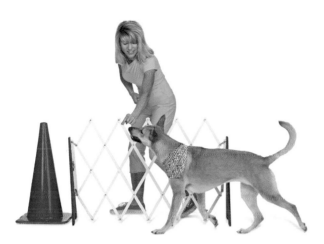

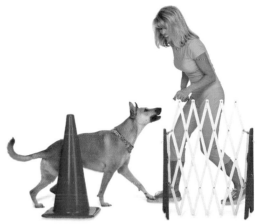

1 Set up a barrel or cone for your dog to go around. Position a fence or small barrier leading up to it. Use a treat to lure your dog down the length of the fence, around the cone, and back up the other side of the fence.

2 Move the fence slightly away from the cone and repeat this exercise. Say, "Go around," and stop your body a little before the cone, so your dog has to do that last part by himself.

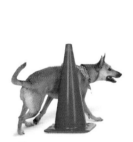

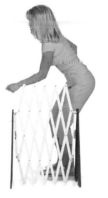

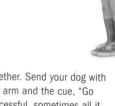

3 Move the fence even farther from the cone. Once your dog has circled the cone, take a step back, so your dog has a little farther to run to get back to you.

4 Finally, remove the fence altogether. Send your dog with an enthusiastic gesture of your arm and the cue, "Go around!" If your dog is not successful, sometimes all it takes is a small bit of fence to remind him what to do.

TIP:	EQUIPMENT:	BUILD ON IT:
If your dog is tagging the cone with his paws instead of circling it, try using a barrel or metal trash can instead.	You need not use an actual barrel to teach this skill. Use any item that is stable and taller than your dog's head, such as a trash can or traffic cone.	Cik & Cap Jump Wraps *page 110*

Fetch

A game of fetch provides hours of entertainment and exercise for you and your dog. (Probably mostly for your dog.)

TEACHING SKILLS:
This fun game teaches a useful retrieve.

PRIMARY USES:

FLYBALL
Flyball is a relay race in which each dog runs down a line of hurdles, grabs a tennis ball at the end and brings it back to the start line.

OBEDIENCE
The dumbbell retrieve is a component in competition obedience.

FIELD RETRIEVING
Sporting dogs are trained to locate and retrieve downed birds. Rubber dummies are often substituted for birds in retrieving competition.

SERVICE DOG
Fetching objects is the most common skill required of a service dog. The dog may fetch a dropped item or item from the next room.

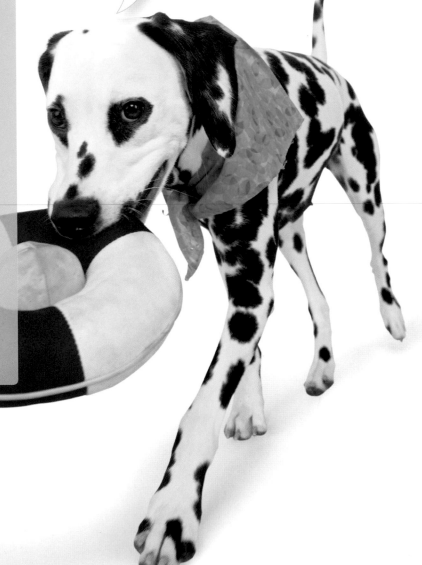

I have so much to do every day I don't know how I can possibly get it all done!

TRY IT:

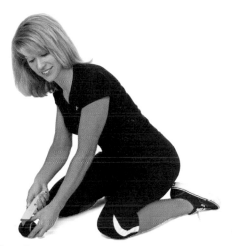

1 Use a box cutter to make a 1-inch (2.5 cm) slit in a tennis ball.

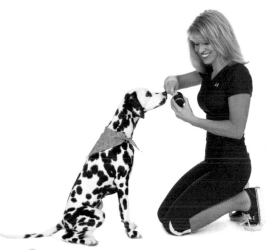

2 Squeeze the ball so the slit opens and show your dog while you drop treats inside.

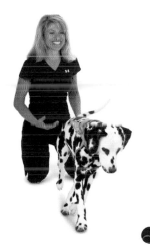

3 Get your dog interested in the ball by bouncing it and batting it around. Toss the ball playfully and encourage your dog to chase it. Try to get him to bring it back to you by patting your legs, acting excited, or running from him.

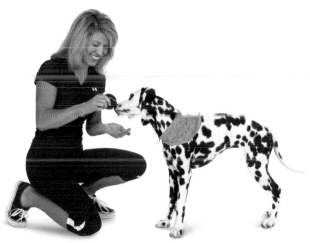

4 When your dog does (eventually) bring the ball back near you, squeeze it to let the treats drop out for him. As your dog is unable to get the treats out for himself, he will quickly learn to bring the ball back to you for his reward.

TIP:

Never chase your dog when he is playing keep-away. Lure him back with a treat or run away from him to encourage him to chase you. Have a second ball to get his attention.

EQUIPMENT:

Used tennis balls can be easily acquired at tennis courts. Excessive mouthing of tennis balls can lead to tooth wear, so if your dog is a chewer, switch to a rubber ball. Choose a ball that is big enough that your dog cannot swallow it and soft enough that it will not break his teeth if he catches it midair.

BUILD ON IT:

Disc Rollers
page 118

Flyball Fetch
page 146

Flyball Fetch

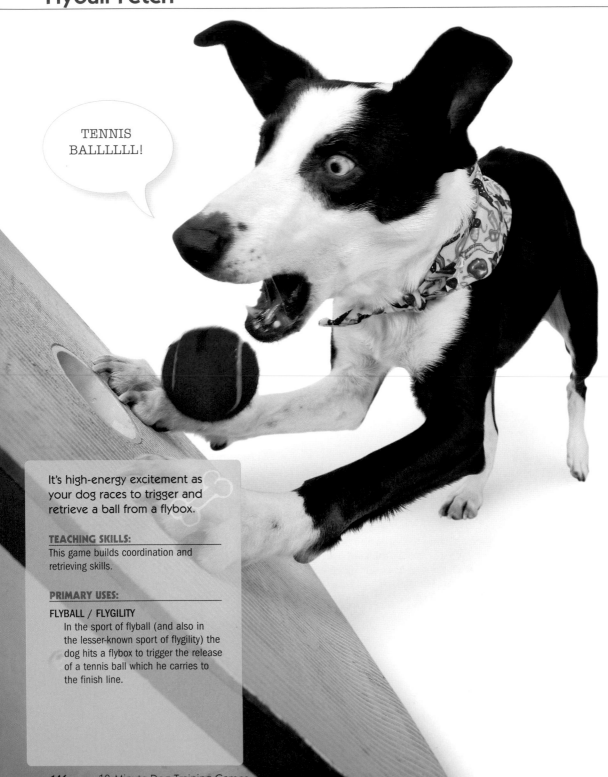

TENNIS BALLLLLL!

It's high-energy excitement as your dog races to trigger and retrieve a ball from a flybox.

TEACHING SKILLS:

This game builds coordination and retrieving skills.

PRIMARY USES:

FLYBALL / FLYGILITY

In the sport of flyball (and also in the lesser-known sport of flygility) the dog hits a flybox to trigger the release of a tennis ball which he carries to the finish line.

TRY IT:

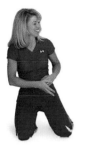
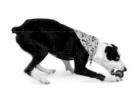
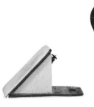
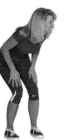
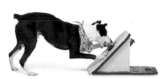

1 First, teach your dog to Fetch (page 144). Toss the tennis ball toward the flybox and have your dog "fetch." Some dogs enjoy fetching, but most dogs will need a treat as a reward.

2 Next, push the ball into the flybox hole. Start your dog from at least 10 feet (3 m) away and enthusiastically send him to "fetch!" If you send him with a lot of energy, he will hopefully jump forcefully on the box and trigger the ball's release.

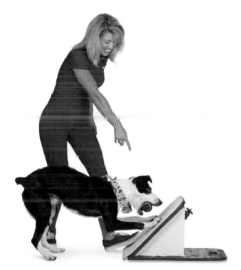
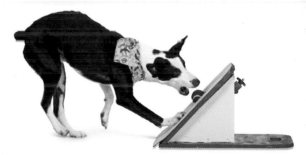

3 If he is not triggering the ball, you are going to have to trigger it for him. Stand close to the flybox, and when your dog touches the flybox at all, press the board with your foot to trigger the ball's release. Praise your dog excitedly so that he thinks HE triggered the ball.

4 Gradually increase the distance so your dog gets to run at top speed to trigger the ball.

TIP:

The trick to teaching this game is to get your dog very excited and running very fast, so that he jumps on the flybox board with enough force to trigger the ball. If your dog scratches at the hole, simply bring him back and try it again.

EQUIPMENT:

A flybox is a slanted box that holds a spring-loaded tennis ball. When the dog hits the box with his front paws, the tennis ball pops out.

BUILD ON IT:

Disc Rollers
page 118

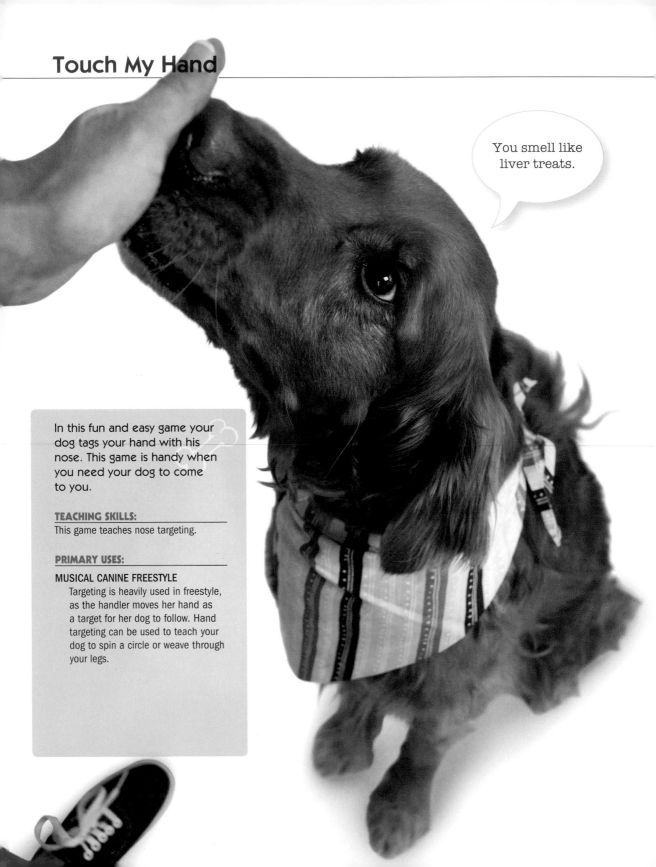

Touch My Hand

You smell like liver treats.

In this fun and easy game your dog tags your hand with his nose. This game is handy when you need your dog to come to you.

TEACHING SKILLS:

This game teaches nose targeting.

PRIMARY USES:

MUSICAL CANINE FREESTYLE
Targeting is heavily used in freestyle, as the handler moves her hand as a target for her dog to follow. Hand targeting can be used to teach your dog to spin a circle or weave through your legs.

TRY IT:

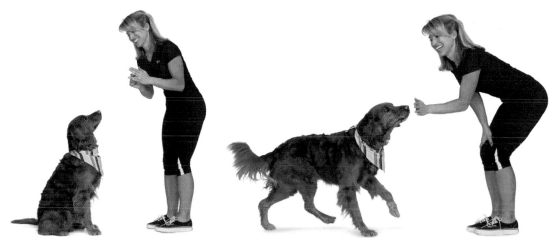

1 Show your dog that you are placing a treat between your fingers.

2 Hold your hand out at your dog's nose height and say, "Touch!" If your dog doesn't notice the treat, wiggle your hand and use your other hand to point to the treat.

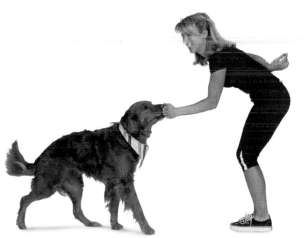

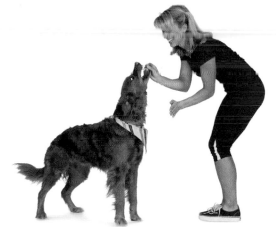

3 The instant your dog's nose touches your hand, say, "Good!" and release the treat.

4 Once your dog gets the hang of this, try it with no treat between your fingers. When your dog touches your hand, say, "Good!" and give him a treat from behind your back.

TIP:

Dogs love this game and catch on quickly. Avoid moving your hand toward your dog's nose, but rather make sure he comes to you.

BUILD ON IT:

Target Stick
page 150

Target Stick

Nose-touching a target stick is a versatile skill with a variety of uses in dog training and dog sports.

TEACHING SKILLS:
This activity teaches targeting skills.

PRIMARY USES:

ANIMAL ACTOR
Target sticks are used by set trainers as a way to move or direct the dog from a distance.

MUSICAL CANINE FREESTYLE
Targeting is heavily used in freestyle. A target stick is used to teach complex moves, such as the dog weaving between the handler's legs.

It's all natural, you know.

TRY IT:

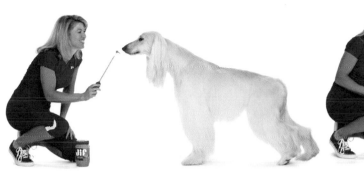

1 Dab a bit of peanut butter on the end of your target stick. Your dog will be tempted to sniff your hand, so hold the stick with the ball more toward your dog. When your dog touches it (with either his nose or tongue), say, "Good!" and give him a treat.

2 After a few repetitions, try it without the peanut butter. The target stick will probably still smell a little like peanut butter, which should be enough to get your dog to sniff it. The instant he touches the target stick say, "Good!" and give him a treat.

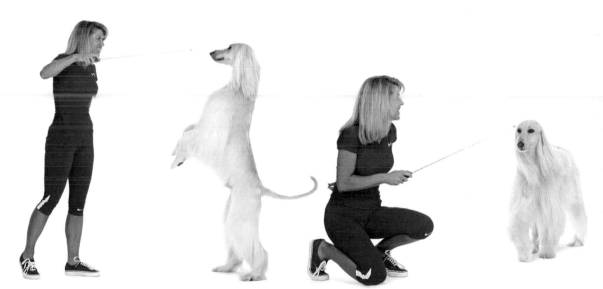

3 Once your dog has the hang of this game, place the target stick at different elevations, both high and low.

4 Have your dog follow a moving target by guiding the target stick away from him.

TIP:	**EQUIPMENT:**	**BUILD ON IT:**
Dogs learn this game pretty quickly and take to it eagerly. The biggest hurdle often is finding the right target stick, which is visible for your dog to see yet not tempting for him to bite.	Professional target sticks are telescoping rods with a small plastic or metal ball at the end. Some target sticks have a clicker on the handle. If you make your own target stick, use a ball on the end that your dog won't be tempted to bite (no tennis balls!).	Paintbrush Painting *page 160*

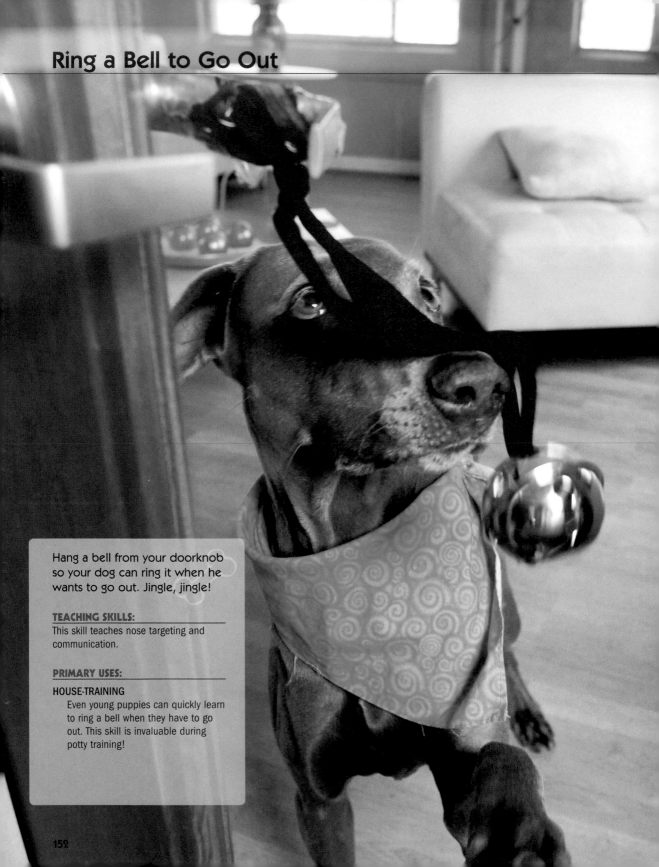

Ring a Bell to Go Out

Hang a bell from your doorknob so your dog can ring it when he wants to go out. Jingle, jingle!

TEACHING SKILLS:
This skill teaches nose targeting and communication.

PRIMARY USES:

HOUSE-TRAINING
Even young puppies can quickly learn to ring a bell when they have to go out. This skill is invaluable during potty training!

TRY IT:

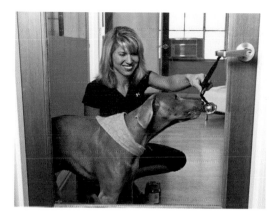

1 Dab a bit of peanut butter on the bell and point it out to your dog. When he goes to sniff it or lick it, use your finger to make it jingle softly.

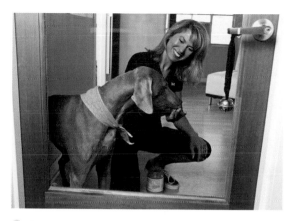

2 Immediately after the jingle, say, "Good!" and give your dog a treat.

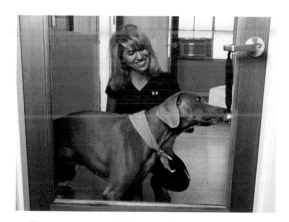

3 After a few repetitions, your dog will probably have licked all of the peanut butter off, but don't add more. Simply touch the bell or point to it and say, "Jingle." Give your dog a treat if he makes it jingle.

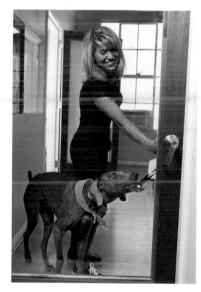

4 Whenever you are about to let your dog outside, have him jingle the bell and then immediately open the door.

TIP:	EQUIPMENT:	BUILD ON IT:
In the beginning, be very responsive to your dog's jingling and open the door for him every time he does it. Dogs, even puppies, catch on pretty quickly and learn to jingle the bell when they need to go out.	Choose a bell large enough that your dog cannot accidentally swallow it. Hang it from the doorknob at your dog's nose height.	Treibball *page 156*

Volleyball

Toss a ball in the air and your dog will bop it back to you with his nose!

TEACHING SKILLS:

This game increases coordination and teaches a nose-touch.

PRIMARY USES:

FLYING DISC
This game teaches your dog the mouth–eye coordination needed to jump and catch a flying disc out of the air.

Watch me bounce it up to the ceiling!

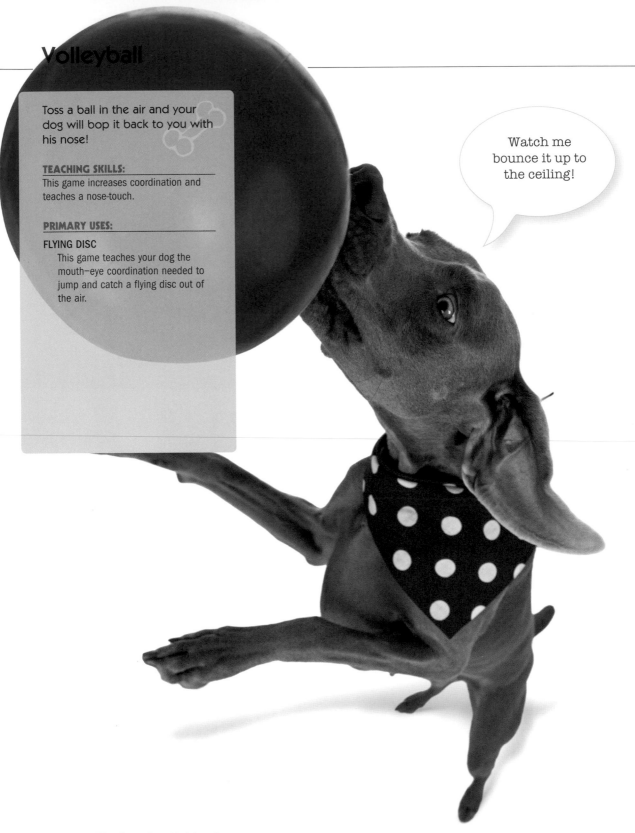

TRY IT:

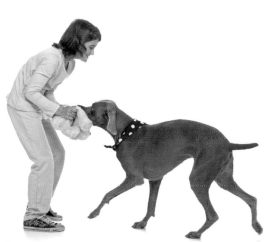

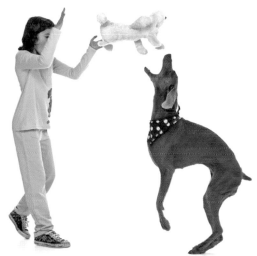

1 Get your dog excited to play with a plush toy. Toss it around and squeak the squeaker to get your dog's interest. Don't push it toward him, but rather draw it away from him to make him chase it.

2 When your dog is focused on the toy, toss it in the air in a slow arc toward him. When he catches it, say, "Good!" and give him a treat.

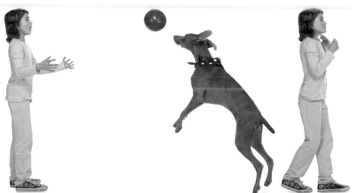

3 While your dog is still feeling playful, switch to a lightweight ball. Toss the ball in a high arc so that it comes down rather vertically above your dog's nose.

4 Because of the large circumference of the ball, your dog will be unable to catch it, and the ball will instead bounce off his nose and back to you!

TIP:	EQUIPMENT:	BUILD ON IT:
This game is often easier than it looks, and your dog could be bouncing a ball off his nose within ten minutes. A balloon will be easier for your dog, as it falls more slowly.	Use a lightweight ball or balloon (be sure to pick up the pieces if the balloon pops so that your dog doesn't eat them). A regulation volleyball will be too heavy for your dog.	Target Stick *page 150*

Treibball

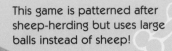

This game is patterned after sheep-herding but uses large balls instead of sheep!

TEACHING SKILLS:

This game teaches a nose touch and improves your dog's coordination.

PRIMARY USES:

TREIBBALL

Treibball (or push ball) is a sport in which a dog maneuvers fitness balls across a field into a goal. It originated as an activity for herding dogs who didn't have access to sheep and large fields. In the same way that a herding dog prods sheep into a pen, he now prods large balls into a goal.

HERDING

Treibball is a quickly growing activity among herding-breed owners as an off-season or indoor substitute for sheep herding.

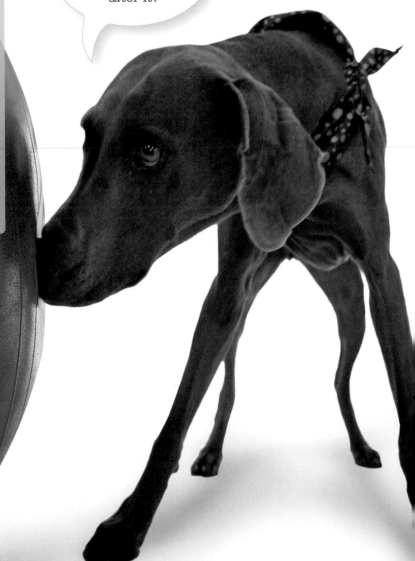

TRY IT:

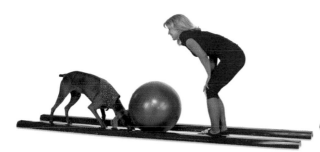

1 Construct a chute for your ball to roll through by setting up two rails or by placing a sofa parallel to a wall. Put the ball at one end of the chute and place a treat at the base of the ball. As your dog reaches for the treat, he will bump the ball forward.

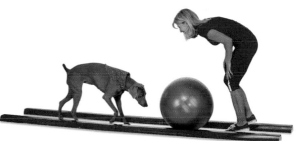

2 Repeat this exercise, but this time set a few additional treats in the chute behind the ball. After your dog bumps the ball, he will see the next treat.

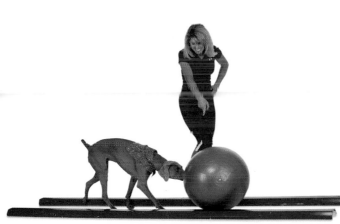

3 Don't set any treats on the floor this time, but encourage your dog to "push!" When he pushes the ball, even a little, say, "Good!" and toss a treat at the base of the ball.

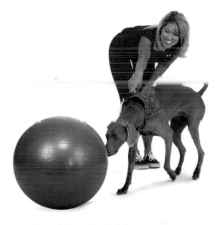

4 Remove the training rails. Wait for your dog to push the ball twice before saying, "Good!" and tossing a treat near the base of the ball.

TIP:	**EQUIPMENT:**	**BUILD ON IT:**
Some dogs will get very excited and bite and pop the ball while learning. It is important to deliver your treat near the base of the ball to encourage your dog to poke under the ball instead of biting it.	Use large 22 to 34-inch (55 to 85 cm) exercise balls. Initial training can done with smaller and more heavy-duty balls (piglet balls, Jolly Balls, Ferkelballs, or Enduro Balls). Training rails can be made from wood beams or rain gutters.	Volleyball *page 154*

Soap Bubbles

Does your dog love to chase soap bubbles? Give it a try and find out!

TEACHING SKILLS:

This game will improve your dog's coordination and nose touch skill.

PRIMARY USES:

FLYING DISC

This game helps your dog develop the mouth-eye coordination needed to catch a flying disc.

TRY IT:

Try this game when your dog is in a playful mood. Blow some bubbles up into the air (not toward your dog) and encourage him to, "Get it! Get it!" Bubbles can be more fun outdoors, as the breeze makes them fly away like insects.

TIP:

Some dogs go nuts for this game! Other dogs have little interest in the bubbles. Oftentimes breeds that were bred to chase small vermin (such as terriers) take most readily to this chase.

EQUIPMENT:

Children's toy soap bubbles are nontoxic and work just fine for dogs. However, specialty meat and peanut-butter-flavored bubbles are also available for dogs!

BUILD ON IT:

Volleyball
page 154

Roll Out the Carpet

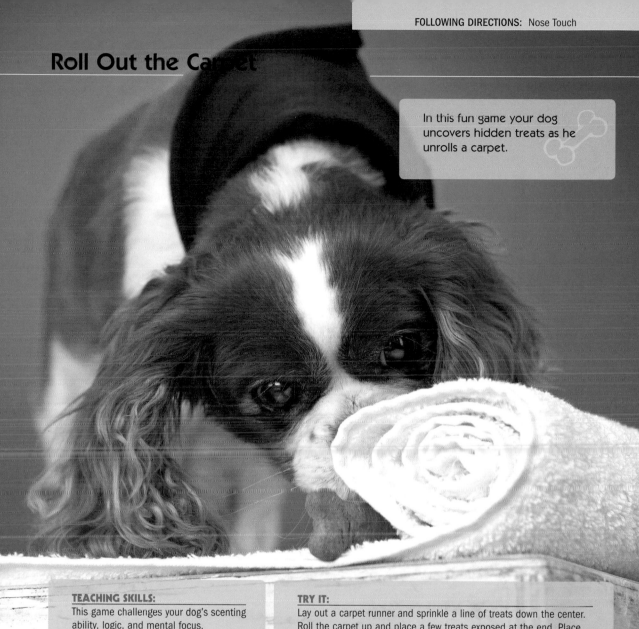

In this fun game your dog uncovers hidden treats as he unrolls a carpet.

TEACHING SKILLS:

This game challenges your dog's scenting ability, logic, and mental focus.

PRIMARY USES:

TRACKING

This game teaches your dog to sniff the ground to detect faint scents. His persistence is rewarded.

TRY IT:

Lay out a carpet runner and sprinkle a line of treats down the center. Roll the carpet up and place a few treats exposed at the end. Place one of the treats wedged under the roll. Point the treats out to your dog and encourage him to "get it!" When he reaches for the treat wedged under the roll, he will end up unrolling the carpet a little, and hopefully exposing another treat. If he didn't unroll it enough to expose a treat, help him by unrolling the carpet a little for him.

EQUIPMENT:

A carpet runner gives your dog a good, long roll; however it may be too heavy for small dogs. A small rug works well, and a bath mat is very light weight and easy to unroll.

BUILD ON IT:

Treibball
page 156

Paintbrush Painting

To all the puppy Pawcassos out there . . . this one's for you!

I maybe went outside the lines a little.

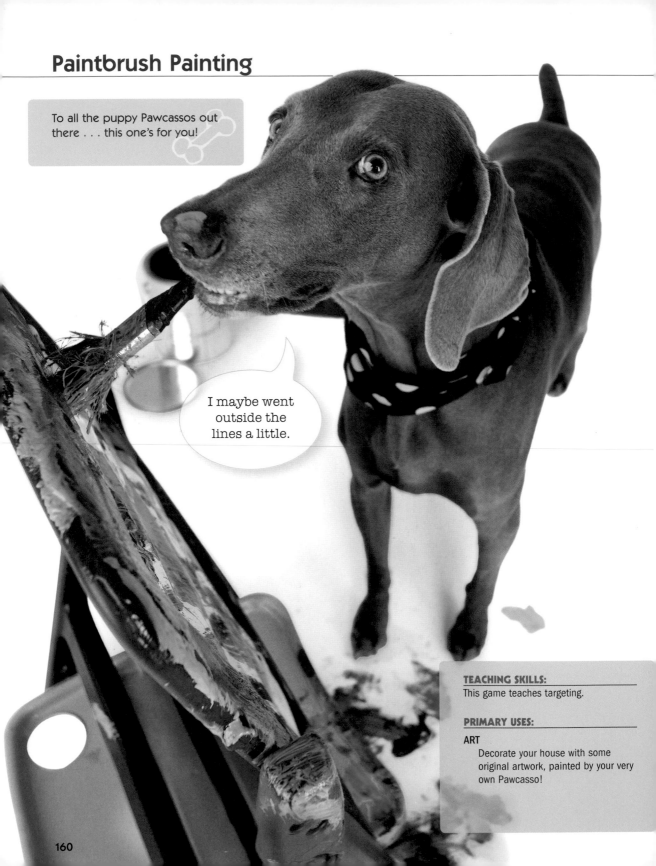

TEACHING SKILLS:
This game teaches targeting.

PRIMARY USES:

ART
Decorate your house with some original artwork, painted by your very own Pawcasso!

TRY IT:

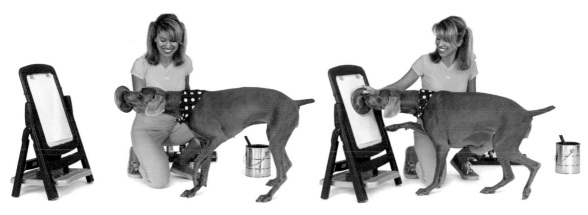

1 First teach your dog Touch My Hand (page 148). Practice having your dog nose-touch a flat object, such as a paint-can lid. You may have to tap the lid or even put a dab of peanut butter on it for the first couple of times.

2 Tape or hold the lid against your easel. Say, "Touch!" and give your dog a treat for nose-touching it.

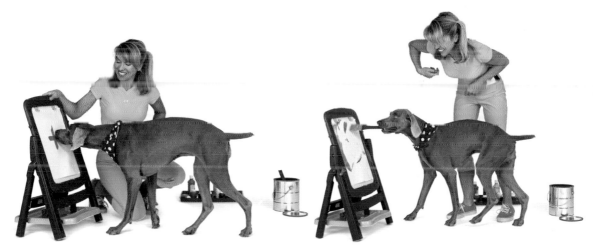

3 Remove the lid and instead use colored tape to mark an X on the canvas. Tap the X and tell your dog to "touch!"

4 Hopefully your dog enjoys holding things in her mouth or has learned to Fetch (page 144). Have her take the paintbrush in her mouth and then cue her to nose-touch the canvas. Because the paintbrush extends in front of her, she will end up stabbing the brush into the easel.

TIP:

Tap the canvas to guide your dog to it, especially if the paintbrush is not perfectly straight in her mouth. Many dogs drop the paintbrush immediately after touching it to the canvas, so you may need to reset the brush after every stroke.

EQUIPMENT:

Use nontoxic, washable kids' paint. A wooden-handled paintbrush will be the most comfortable for your dog to hold.

BUILD ON IT:

Pawprint Painting
page 170

Tennis Ball in Sandbox

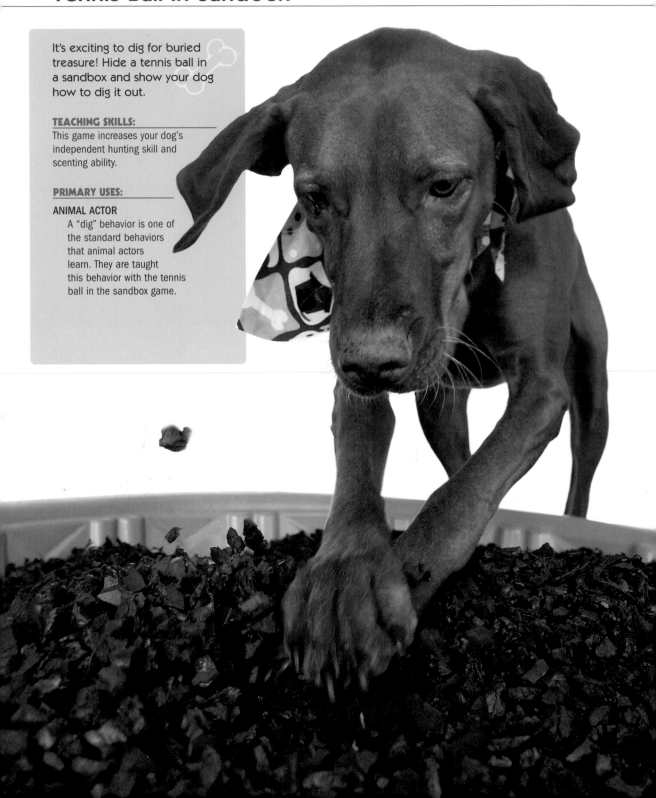

It's exciting to dig for buried treasure! Hide a tennis ball in a sandbox and show your dog how to dig it out.

TEACHING SKILLS:

This game increases your dog's independent hunting skill and scenting ability.

PRIMARY USES:

ANIMAL ACTOR
A "dig" behavior is one of the standard behaviors that animal actors learn. They are taught this behavior with the tennis ball in the sandbox game.

TRY IT:

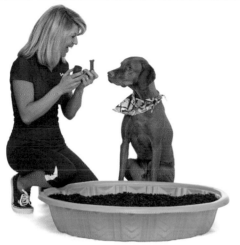

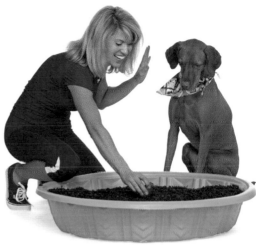

1 Hide a treat inside a ventilated canister or cut a 1-inch (2.5 cm) slit in a tennis ball and hide a treat inside it. Let your dog watch you and sniff the canister.

2 Bury the canister just barely under the surface and maybe even partially visible.

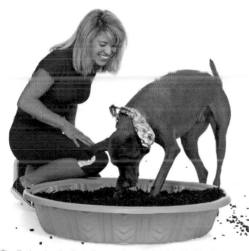

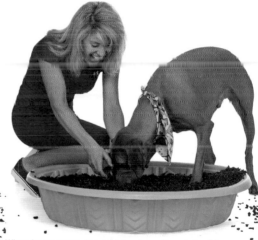

3 Enthusiastically tell your dog, "Dig! Dig!" If he is hesitant, pull the canister out, let him sniff it, and bury it again.

4 When he uncovers the canister, open it and give him the treat near the spot where he found it (it will increase the excitement of the game if he feels as if he dug up the treat).

TIP:

If your dog tries to nose for the canister instead of digging, cover the canister for a second with your hand and then give him the idea to dig by digging a little yourself with your hand.

EQUIPMENT:

Rubber mulch, sold at gardening stores, is a cleaner substitute for real dirt or sand. A baby food jar with ventilation holes punched in the lid works as a canister.

BUILD ON IT:

Treat under a Blanket
page 37

Wipe Your Paws
page 164

Wipe Your Paws

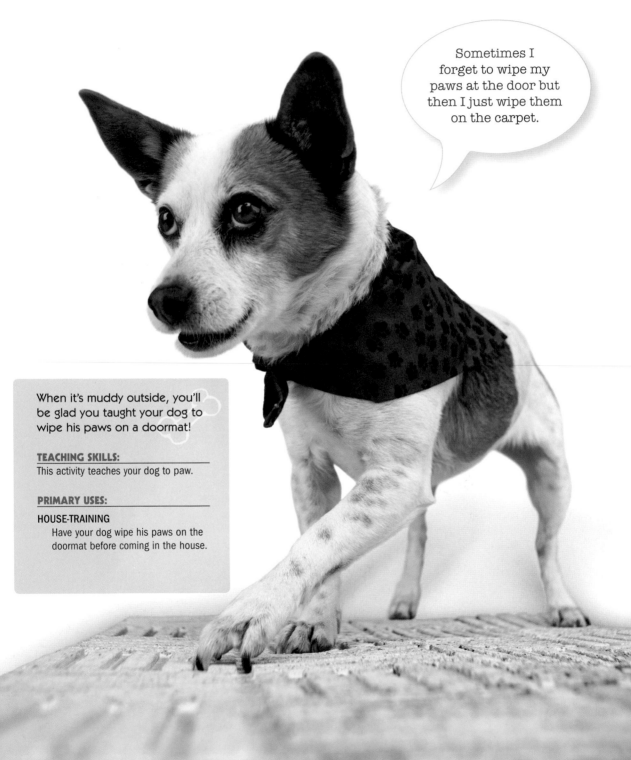

Sometimes I forget to wipe my paws at the door but then I just wipe them on the carpet.

When it's muddy outside, you'll be glad you taught your dog to wipe his paws on a doormat!

TEACHING SKILLS:

This activity teaches your dog to paw.

PRIMARY USES:

HOUSE-TRAINING

Have your dog wipe his paws on the doormat before coming in the house.

TRY IT:

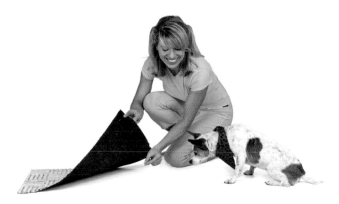

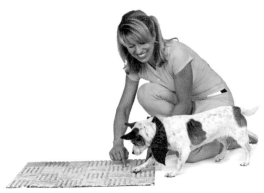

1 Show your dog as you put a treat on the ground (hard dog biscuits work best). Cover the treat with the doormat, so that the treat is near the corner of the mat.

2 Hold the edge of the doormat down, because your dog will probably try to poke his nose under it. Keep encouraging your dog, "Get it! Get it!" If he loses interest, quickly lift the corner of the doormat to show him the treat and put it back down again.

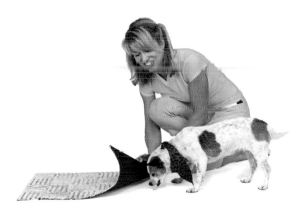

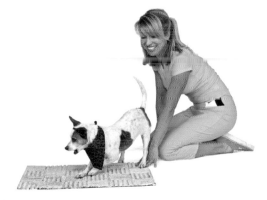

3 When he gets frustrated, your dog will scratch at the doormat—be ready for this! The instant he does even one scratch, say, "Good!" and lift the doormat for him to get the treat.

4 As he gets better, wait for him to do two or three scratches before rewarding him. You can then stop putting the treat under the doormat and toss it where he is digging instead (it will be more fun for him if he "digs up" the treat rather than getting it from your hand).

TIP:	**EQUIPMENT:**	**BUILD ON IT:**
Dogs enjoy this game and the excitement of "digging up" their treat. Dogs usually nose the doormat a lot at first and might do just one tentative scratch—don't miss it! Reward your dog for just the slightest scratch, and in no time he'll be wiping his paws like a good dog!	Your dog will be scratching the mat (as opposed to gently wiping his paws), so choose a fairly heavy-duty mat that won't rip and won't bunch up.	Scratchy Board *page 166* Scratch Art *page 168*

Scratchy Board

If your dog dislikes having his nails trimmed, teach him to file his own nails by scratching at a sandpaper board.

TEACHING SKILLS:
This teaches a pawing behavior.

PRIMARY USES:

NAIL TRIMMING
Many dogs dislike having their paws handled and their nails trimmed. With this game, your dog scratches at an abrasive surface to trim his own nails. Some dogs (particularly terriers) enjoy it so much that their owners must hide the scratchy board from their dog.

I don't like having my nails trimmed so I usually kick a lot or run away.

TRY IT:

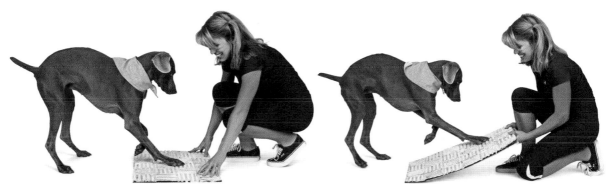

1 First teach your dog Wipe Your Paws (page 164). Next, lay the doormat on top of the scratchy board on the floor, and have your dog wipe his paws. Give him a treat for doing so.

2 Raise one end of the board and doormat slightly. Sit near the high end of the board and try to get your dog to scratch again. When you reward him, do so by tossing the treat on the high end of the doormat, because your dog will focus on the place where the treat appears.

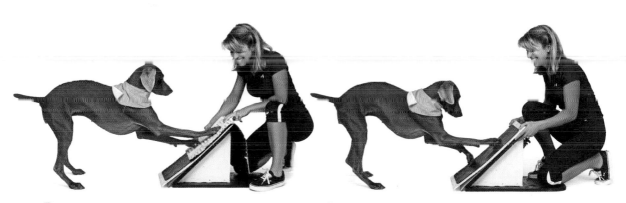

3 Partially slide the doormat off the top end of the board and raise the angle a bit more. Your dog will scratch at the doormat, but his paws will sometimes also end up brushing against the scratchy board.

4 Keep sliding the doormat up, until it is entirely gone. Tell your dog, "Scratch! Scratch!" and tap the scratchy board occasionally to keep him focused. Periodically give him a treat near the top of the board.

TIP:	EQUIPMENT:	BUILD ON IT:
Some dogs find this game self-rewarding and will do it even without a treat. If your dog is a tenacious scratcher, you may need to hide the scratchy board away when you are not home.	Affix sandpaper to a sturdy board using a staple gun or glue.	Scratch Art *page 168*

Scratch Art

Turn your dog's scratching skill into art by using scratch art paper.

TEACHING SKILLS:
This art project uses pawing skills.

PRIMARY USES:

ART
Decorate your house with some original artwork, scratched just for you!

TRY IT:
Teach your dog Wipe Your Paws (page 164). Have him scratch the doormat a few times for practice. Then lay your scratch art paper (attached to a clipboard) on top of where he was scratching and cue him again. *Voilà!* Art!

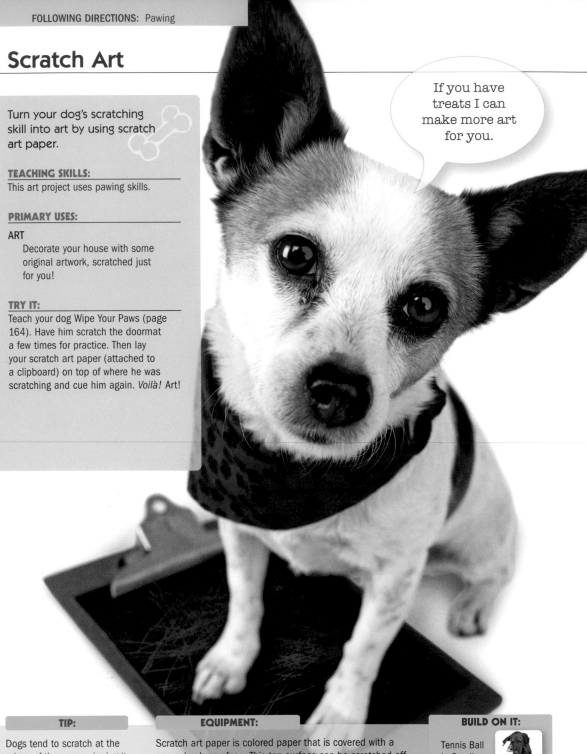

If you have treats I can make more art for you.

TIP:

Dogs tend to scratch at the edges of the paper, ripping it. You may have to tape down the edges to a clipboard.

EQUIPMENT:

Scratch art paper is colored paper that is covered with a second color surface. This top surface can be scratched off to reveal the color below. You can get a similar effect using transfer paper (such as carbon paper). Since transfer paper is thin, cover the sheets in plastic page protectors.

BUILD ON IT:

Tennis Ball in Sandbox *page 162*

Test Right- or Left-Pawed

This is my good one.

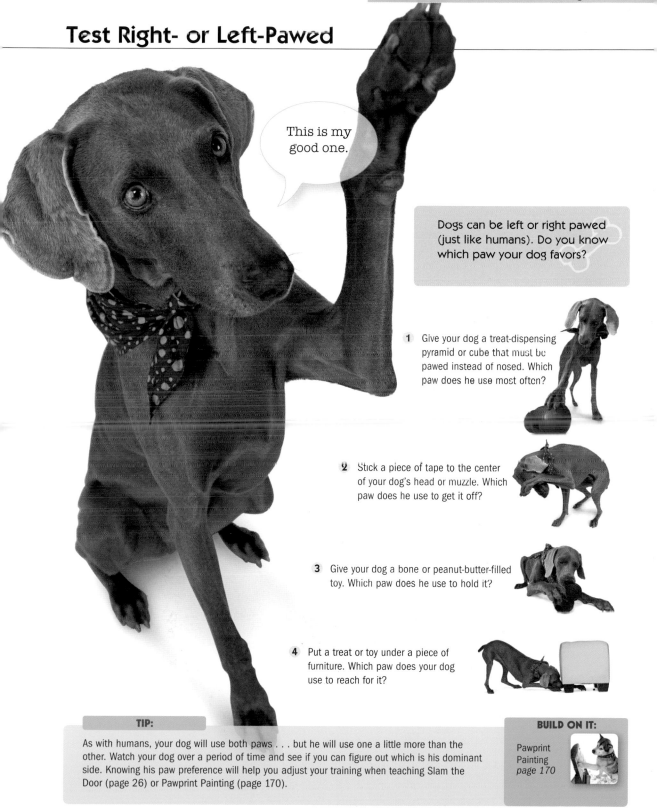

Dogs can be left or right pawed (just like humans). Do you know which paw your dog favors?

1 Give your dog a treat-dispensing pyramid or cube that must be pawed instead of nosed. Which paw does he use most often?

2 Stick a piece of tape to the center of your dog's head or muzzle. Which paw does he use to get it off?

3 Give your dog a bone or peanut-butter-filled toy. Which paw does he use to hold it?

4 Put a treat or toy under a piece of furniture. Which paw does your dog use to reach for it?

TIP:

As with humans, your dog will use both paws . . . but he will use one a little more than the other. Watch your dog over a period of time and see if you can figure out which is his dominant side. Knowing his paw preference will help you adjust your training when teaching Slam the Door (page 26) or Pawprint Painting (page 170).

BUILD ON IT:

Pawprint Painting
page 170

Pawprint Painting

Help your dog create a work of art as he spreads paint on canvas with his paws. So cute!

TEACHING SKILLS:
This activity is a pawing skill.

Shoot! Ripped another one.

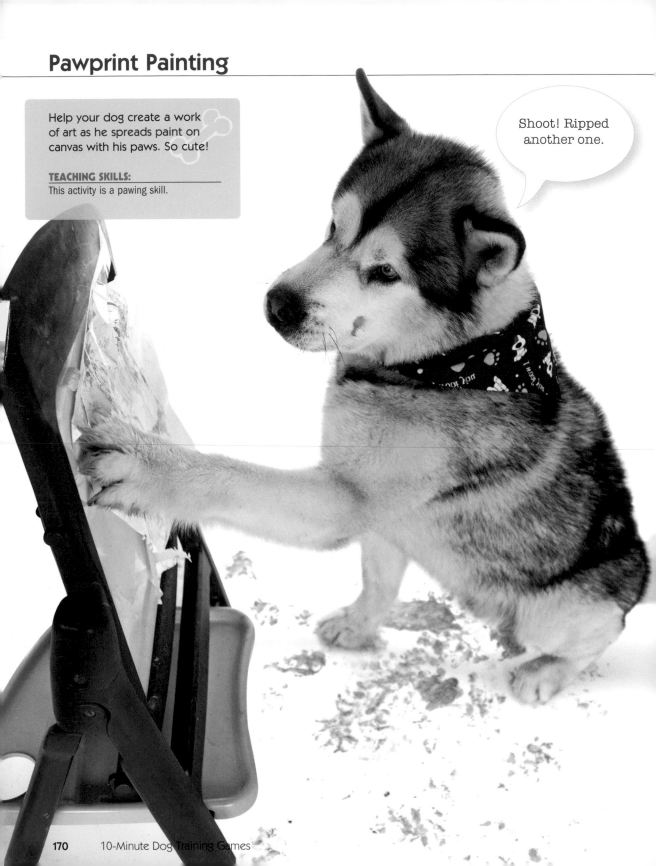

TRY IT:

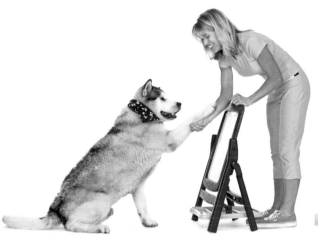

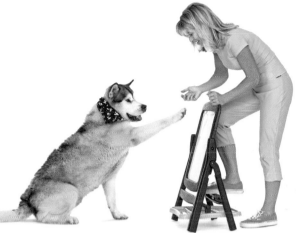

1   For the first step, you want your dog to give you his paw. If he knows a cue word for "shake hands," then use that. If not, try holding a treat in your fist, low to the ground, and opening your hand when your dog paws at it.

2   Next, ask your dog to "shake hands," but at the last second, pull your hand back so he is pawing at the air, or even at the easel. Give him a treat for this.

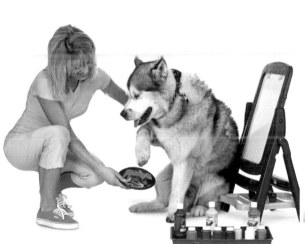

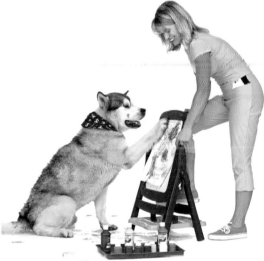

3   Pour some paint into a plate, lift your dog's paw, and press the paint onto his paw (and not his paw down into the paint).

4   Stand behind the easel, hold out your hand, and ask your dog to shake hands. Again, pull your hand out of the way so he paws at the paper. Give him a treat each time that he does!

TIP:	EQUIPMENT:	BUILD ON IT:
Do your painting outdoors or in the shower. Have your dog lay down one color and let it dry for a minute before laying down the next color (otherwise it can turn into a muddy-colored mess). It may be easier to lay the easel in your lap.	Use nontoxic, washable kids' paint.	Paintbrush Painting *page 160*

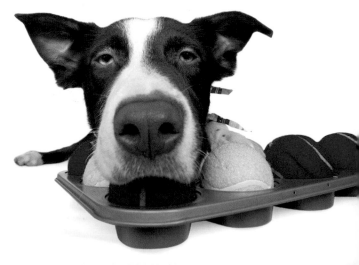

INDEX BY SPORT

ACKNOWLEDGMENTS

Thanks to **Heidi Horn** (production assistant, dog wrangler, bandanna coordinator, and dog petter), **Kylie Horn** (child supermodel), **Claire Doré** (dog wrangler), and my own Weimaraners **Chalcy** and **Jadie**. Thanks to all the beautiful and talented dogs who participated in the photo shoots: **Skippy** (Jack Russell terrier), **Iris** (terrier mix), **Owen** (golden retriever), **Lola** (long-haired Chihuahua), **Laci** (Dalmatian), **Duke** (vizsla), **Caesar** (standard poodle), **Elliott** (Australian shepherd), **Dakota** (Labrador retriever), **Charlie** (Afghan hound), **Jackson** (yellow shepherd mix), **Kwin** and **Jeep** (Alaskan malamutes), **Lassie** (rough collie), **Flash** and **Torch** (McNabs), **Fiona** (Irish wolfhound), **Drover** (Brittany), and **Conner** (cavalier King Charles spaniel). Thanks to **FitPAWS** dog balance balls.

PHOTOGRAPHY

and toy squeaking by Christian Arias, Slickforce Studios, www.slickforce.com

IN MEMORIAM: Before this book went to print, one of its very special dogs passed away. Alaskan malamute "**Jeep**" (page 47) was an outgoing girl with a promising future in competition obedience and dog mushing. She loved to romp in the outdoors and chase radio-controlled cars. Jeep suffered from uncontrollable epilepsy and seizures. Our dogs fill our hearts when they are with us and then, for a while, our hearts are broken when they leave us. But they will always live on in our hearts, in a space reserved just for them.

 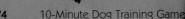

101 DOG TRICKS

STEP-BY-STEP ACTIVITIES TO ENGAGE, CHALLENGE, AND BOND WITH YOUR DOG

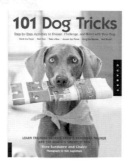

This international bestseller is the industry standard training book for adult dogs. Difficulty ratings range from "easy" to "expert" and "build-on" ideas suggest more complicated tricks that build on each new skill. If you want to teach your dog to *find the remote, carry your purse, play basketball,* and *jump rope,* then this is the book for you!

THE DOG TRICKS AND TRAINING WORKBOOK

A STEP-BY-STEP INTERACTIVE CURRICULUM TO ENGAGE, CHALLENGE, AND BOND WITH YOUR DOG

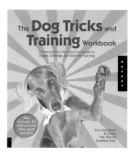

Track your progress as you work through this comprehensive curriculum. *Review* and *re-evaluation* sections at the end of each chapter prompt you to reflect on your progress and your improving relationship with your dog. *It also includes* 30 trick cards and a DVD.

51 PUPPY TRICKS

STEP-BY-STEP ACTIVITIES TO ENGAGE, CHALLENGE, AND BOND WITH YOUR PUPPY

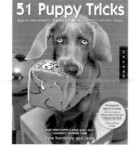

By teaching your puppy early and using positive reinforcement methods, you will instill in her a cooperative spirit and a lifetime love of learning. Especially for puppies ages birth to two years. It includes *ring a bell to go out, loose-leash walk, wipe your paws,* and *fetch.*

101 WAYS TO DO MORE WITH YOUR DOG!

MAKE YOUR DOG A SUPERDOG WITH SPORTS, GAMES, EXERCISES, TRICKS, MENTAL CHALLENGES, CRAFTS, BONDING

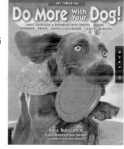

Learn about agility, dock diving, dog dancing, therapy visits, doga, nose-work, tracking . . . and more. With 101 dog sports and activities to choose from, you're sure to find some that inspire you and your dog.

BEST OF 101 DOG TRICKS (DVD)
BEST PUPPY TRICKS (DVD)

STARRING KYRA SUNDANCE

These award-winning DVDs feature step-by-step instruction and real-world examples of training a novice dog. The **Puppy Tricks DVD** contains 17 tricks including *Spin Circles, Open the Door, Close the Door, Roll Over, Ring a Bell to Go Outside, Wipe Your Paws, Turn on the Tap Light,* and *Fetch.* The **Dog Tricks DVD** contains 16 tricks including *Say Your Prayers, Jump through My Circled Arms, Shake Hands, Crawl, Beg, Take a Bow, Cover Your Eyes,* and *Tidy Up Your Toys.*

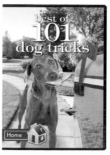
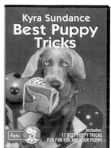

ABOUT THE AUTHOR

KYRA SUNDANCE is a world-acclaimed professional stunt dog show performer, a nationally ranked dog sports competitor, and internationally best-selling author. Comprising the Sundance Dog Team, Kyra and her precision-trained Weimaraners have starred in a command performance for the king of Morocco in Marrakech, in Disney's *Underdog* stage show in Hollywood, in the *Showdog Moms & Dads* television series, and in circuses and sports halftime shows internationally. They have performed on *The Tonight Show*, *Ellen*, *Entertainment Tonight*, the *Worldwide Fido Awards*, and on Animal Planet.

Kyra set trains dog actors for TV and movies including *Beverly Hills Chihuahua 2*. She competes in a variety of dog sports and holds national ranking. Kyra lectures internationally on positive training techniques for professional organizations such as APDT, CAPPDT, and IACP.

Kyra's many popular dog-training books and DVDs include the international bestseller *101 Dog Tricks* and the award-winning *Best of Dog Tricks* DVD series. Kyra holds the human-dog bond at the heart of her training method. She cares for her dogs with tenderness, trains them thoroughly, and inspires them to excel. Her methods foster confident, happy dogs who are motivated to do the right thing rather than ones fearful of making a mistake. She shows us how to develop joyful relationships with dogs who balance enthusiasm with self-control.

Kyra is a UCLA alumnus, marathon runner, and former Club Med windsurfing instructor. She lives with her Weimaraners and her husband, Randy Banis, on their ranch in California's Mojave Desert.

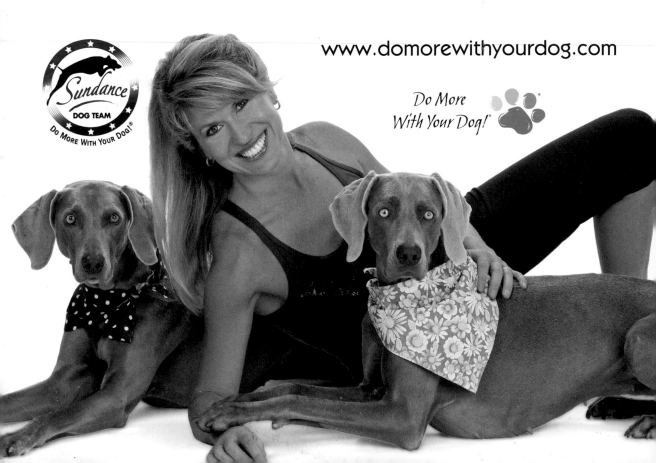

www.domorewithyourdog.com

Sundance
DOG TEAM
DO MORE WITH YOUR DOG!®

Do More With Your Dog!®